PRAISE FOR
REGENERATIVE PERFOMANCE

"Having *Regenerative Performance* in your hands is like having your own personal performance coach in your pocket. This isn't about quick fixes or rigid routines—it's about breaking free from the cycle of burnout and learning how to excel without sacrificing well-being."

—TOMMY HUGHES, HEAD OF PEOPLE PERFORMANCE, ASTON MARTIN ARAMCO FORMULA ONE® TEAM

"A game-changing blueprint for sustainable high performance. James Hewitt's Cognitive Gears model—viewing knowledge work as an endurance sport—is a standout concept that leaders can immediately apply to themselves and their teams."

—MARK KELLY, GLOBAL HEAD OF BENEFITS & WELLBEING, BOSTON CONSULTING GROUP

"Whether you're an executive, entrepreneur, or high-achiever looking for a better way, *Regenerative Performance* offers a blueprint for sustainable success that won't leave you drained and depleted."

—JOSH LINKNER, FIVE-TIME TECH ENTREPRENEUR, *NEW YORK TIMES* BESTSELLING AUTHOR, AND VENTURE CAPITALIST

"James Hewitt brings the heavy artillery of data analysis and deeply understood medical research to blast away at pseudoscientific narratives."

—ERIC SCHURENBERG, FORMER CEO OF INC. AND FAST COMPANY

"*Regenerative Performance* gives us the road map, grounded in science, to reframe stress and overload so that we can sustainably thrive."

—DR. NATALIE NIXON, AUTHOR OF *MOVE. THINK. REST.*

"Be warned that this book comes with a 'health warning': this book will change your life—for the better!"

—HARRI SUNDVIK, FORMER VICE CHAIR OF BANK OF AMERICA

"James has been a guest on my podcast multiple times, and one of my favorite quotes from him remains: 'People tend to major in the minors; we need to major in the majors.' This book does exactly that—helping us focus on what truly matters for sustainable performance and health."

—GREG BENNETT, OLYMPIAN, FORMER WORLD NUMBER ONE TRIATHLETE, ENTREPRENEUR, AND HOST OF *THE GREG BENNETT SHOW*

REGENERATIVE PERFORMANCE

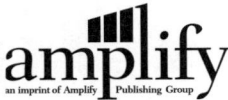

amplify
an imprint of Amplify | Publishing Group

www.amplifypublishinggroup.com

Regenerative Performance: How to Thrive in an Always-On World Without Sacrificing Your Well-Being

This book is not intended as a substitute for the medical advice of physicians. The reader should regularly consult a physician in matters relating to their health and particularly with respect to any symptoms that may require diagnosis or medical attention.

For more information, please contact:
Amplify Publishing, an imprint of Amplify Publishing Group
620 Herndon Parkway, Suite 220
Herndon, VA 20170
info@amplifypublishing.com

Library of Congress Control Number: 2025905149

CPSIA Code: PRV0425A

ISBN-13: 979-8-89138-486-6

Printed in the United States

To Anna, whose love and support made this book possible, and to everyone seeking a more sustainable path to extraordinary performance.

DR. JAMES HEWITT

REGENERATIVE PERFORMANCE

HOW TO THRIVE IN AN ALWAYS-ON WORLD WITHOUT SACRIFICING YOUR WELL-BEING

amplify

CONTENTS

FOREWORD

BY SIR CLIVE WOODWARD

When James first introduced me to the concept of Regenerative Performance, it struck a chord immediately. Over the years, working with world-class teams in rugby and Olympic sport, I've learned that high performance isn't just about pushing harder and working longer; it's about sustaining excellence under pressure. And that's exactly what this brilliant book is about.

In elite sport, we've long known that success isn't simply about out-working the opposition. Of course, hard work is essential, but the best teams don't just grind; they know when to switch on and when to switch off. They don't just train harder; they train smarter. That's what set the England team apart in the buildup to our Rugby World Cup victory in 2003. We understood that sustained performance required a balance between effort and recovery. The ability to be at your sharpest when it mattered most was our competitive advantage.

The same principles held true when I worked with Team GB at the London 2012 Olympics. The most successful athletes weren't necessarily those who trained the longest hours but those who optimized their energy, their mindset, and their recovery. They had a rhythm to their performance, a discipline in how they prepared, competed, and recovered. That's what James calls Regenerative Performance—an approach that ensures you stay at your best when the stakes are highest.

What makes this brilliant book so powerful is its relevance beyond sport. Today's business world is relentless. Leaders and teams are constantly connected, managing multiple demands, and feeling the pressure to always be "on." But as James rightly points out, high performance isn't about constant intensity; it's about the ability to recover, reset, and go again. That's not just a sports science principle; it's a winning mindset.

James brings a unique perspective to this subject. His background as a racing cyclist, combined with his expertise in performance science, gives him an incredible depth of insight. But what makes his work truly stand out is his brilliant personal journey. His experience battling cancer gave him a profound understanding of resilience, recovery, and what it really takes to sustain performance over the long term.

The strategies outlined in this book are not theoretical; they are practical, proven, and backed by science. Whether you're leading a team, growing a business, or striving for personal excellence, the insights here will help you operate at your best without burning out.

In sport, we talk about marginal gains—what I call doing one hundred things 1 percent better—tiny yet crucial adjustments that collectively make a significant impact. But what James presents here goes beyond that. This is about fundamentally rethinking the way we approach performance. It's about understanding the natural rhythms of effort and recovery, and using them to your advantage.

In an era where burnout is becoming the norm and work-life boundaries are blurred, this brilliant book provides a much-needed roadmap for achieving sustained success. It's a must-read for anyone serious about performing at their best without compromising their health, energy, or long-term potential.

PROLOGUE

I used to believe that life could be optimized like a mathematical equation.

In the early 2000s, I spent several years living in the South of France, racing full-time, pursuing my dream of becoming a professional cyclist.

I wasn't the most talented athlete, so I tried to compensate with data. I quantified, analyzed, and optimized every watt of power output, gram of equipment, and second of recovery. The sport's inherent measurability fed my perfectionist nature, and I pursued every legal advantage with scientific precision.

Ultimately, my cycling career never reached the heights that I hoped for, but it embedded a powerful operating system in my mind: quantification + optimization = success. In the years that followed, this algorithm seemed to work. By my thirties, I had checked off many of the boxes for conventional success—a C-suite position at a promising human performance start-up, a loving family, and a beautiful home. The equation appeared solved.

Then came the morning that shattered my carefully constructed reality. A shower. A lump. A diagnosis that rewrote everything.

Cancer doesn't respect optimization algorithms. Chemotherapy cares nothing for morning routines or blocked-out periods of deep work. The treatment that saved my life stripped away many of my meticulously designed timetables. To put the icing on the cake, our start-up's funding began to falter just as a global pandemic locked down the world.

Lying in a chemotherapy ward, watching poison drip through my veins, I was forced to confront an uncomfortable truth: My optimization obsession was less about peak performance and more about the illusion of control. But giving up wasn't an option—I had a family depending on me, a mortgage to pay, a life to live. I needed what I came to call a third way.

This third way wouldn't abandon science or intentional living, but it would embrace flexibility over rigid optimization. Instead of comparing each day to some idealized peak, it would start with an honest assessment of available resources. Rather than detailed protocols, it would rely on adaptable principles. Most importantly, it would accept that life's greatest challenges rarely arrive on schedule.

I recovered fully, thankfully. But the journey transformed more than my health—it revolutionized my entire philosophy of performance and human potential. I call it Regenerative Performance, a framework born from the crucible of crisis that offers a different path to excellence.

This path begins with a troubling question: Why, despite unprecedented investment in self-improvement and optimization over the past two decades, do surveys show life satisfaction hovering near historic lows? The answer isn't simple, but understanding it is crucial for anyone seeking sustainable success in an increasingly uncertain world.

To explore this territory, we'll need to adopt what the Japanese call shoshin—the beginner's mind. This state of open curiosity, unburdened by expertise or expectation, allows us to see old problems with fresh eyes. It's an approach that served me well when hyperoptimization failed, and it will guide us through the chapters ahead.

My story is just one data point in a larger pattern. As we explore that pattern together, you'll discover why the traditional paths to peak performance are failing so many people—and, more importantly, how to forge your own third way forward.

Welcome to the journey.

CHAPTER 1

REGENERATIVE MORNINGS: IS THERE A RIGHT WAY TO START THE DAY?

What fuels the self-improvement world's fixation on early rising and elaborate morning routines?

Hollywood star Mark Wahlberg gave a behind-the-scenes look at his morning routine in a now-famous social media post.

His day began at 2:30 a.m., with thirty minutes of prayer, followed by an intense workout, a shower, a round of golf, and two meals—yes, two—all before 8:00 a.m.

The response? Equal parts fascination, skepticism, and bemusement. Some were convinced this predawn routine was the key to success. Others didn't believe it was possible for a human to wake up this early. Many simply sat back and watched as the competing camps tore each other apart in the comment section.

Our preoccupation with early rising is nothing new. For centuries, waking before dawn has symbolized discipline and productivity. In 1735 Benjamin Franklin famously wrote, "Early to bed and early to rise makes a man healthy, wealthy, and wise."[1] By Wahlberg's standards, Franklin rose at the leisurely hour of 5:00 a.m. Still, his capacity to wear countless hats—scientist, publisher, revolutionary, diplomat, and inventor, to name just a few—is often credited to his presunrise starts.

But should we all follow Wahlberg's example or Franklin's wisdom and set our alarms for the crack of dawn? In a word, no.

The belief that waking up early inevitably leads to virtue and productivity rests more on puritanical beliefs, anecdotes, and assumptions than evidence.

Individual differences in genetically encoded, biologically driven circadian clocks and sleep regulation mechanisms mean there is no single best way to start the day.[2,3] Rather than fixating on someone else's routine, I encourage you to read this chapter with a shoshin-inspired beginner's mind—with curiosity and openness to discover what might work best for you.

How Hyperoptimization Gurus Tell You to Start Your Day

To be fair, Mark Wahlberg never claimed his extreme morning routine was for everyone, but many took it that way. Since his infamous post, the pressure to follow rigorous morning rituals has only intensified. The most popular ideas have coalesced into a hyperoptimizer playbook for starting your day. It goes something like this:

1. **Wake up early:** Set your alarm for 5:00 a.m. (or ideally earlier)—they consider this essential for success.
2. **Leap out of bed:** Hitting snooze is the cardinal sin of self-improvement—proof, somehow, that we are not worthy.
3. **Seek sunlight:** Head directly into morning sunlight (relocate to the West Coast of North America if necessary).
4. **Delay caffeine:** Don't even think about starting your day with a coffee. The gurus will use persuasive neuroscientific jargon to persuade you to wait 90 to 120 minutes before your first caffeine hit.
5. **Take an ice bath:** Replace coffee with a cold plunge—they'll give you another convincing-sounding neuroscience lesson to explain why this is a good idea.
6. **Prevaricate about breakfast:** After the freezing bath, hyperoptimization gurus may or may not advocate eating breakfast (even they haven't figured that one out yet).

And if you find this routine too difficult? They'll just tell you you're not trying hard enough.

These Hyperoptimized Routines Often Do Not Work

I've run workshops and delivered keynotes all over the world, and I've heard similar stories countless times. People read a book, listen to a few podcasts, follow some influencers, and become convinced that a variation of this morning routine will work for them.

For some people, it does, but we tend to overindex on success stories because of survivorship bias—our inclination to fixate on the accounts of people who experienced positive outcomes while overlooking those who did not.

Success stories are further amplified by confirmation bias—the idea of a rigid morning routine leading to achievement supports our existing beliefs about early rising and socially desirable qualities such as self-discipline.

Finally, neuro-jargon-packed protocols leverage shiny object syndrome— our tendency to place undue attention on new ideas.

Stories that rarely get shared on social media are from the countless number of people who fall into an all-too-familiar triangular relapse pattern.

1. **Initiation:** We're inspired to begin a hyperoptimized morning routine with high motivation and commit to ambitious goals.
2. **Maintenance:** We experience initial enthusiasm, but the rigidity of the routine and the unpredictability of life make it difficult to stick to daily.
3. **Setback:** Sustaining the effort becomes exhausting, leading to setbacks. Motivation wanes, and we return to old habits, such as starting our day by scrolling on our phones, often accompanied by feelings of guilt and failure.

Triangular Relapse Pattern

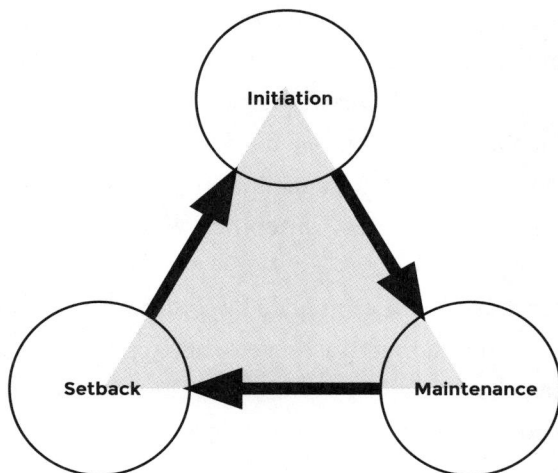

We may try to reboot the routine again in a few weeks or months but often find ourselves oscillating somewhere between superdisciplined *hyperoptimization* or the *quiet quitting* of resignation.

There's a smarter approach—one that steers clear of extreme hyperoptimization and defeatist quiet quitting. But to find it, we need to debunk some common myths, freeing you to design a morning routine that truly works for you.

Unpacking the Truth Behind Popular Claims

Later in the chapter, you'll see that I've devoted significant portions to exploring two specific practices—delaying caffeine in the morning and deliberate cold exposure (cold plunging). My reasoning is twofold. First, these practices are increasingly popular aspects of morning routines being promoted all over the internet. Second, they are both revealing examples of how *hyperoptimizing* influencers present compelling-sounding arguments to support their recommendations when, in fact, many of these arguments are incorrect and clouded by cognitive biases.

Unpacking the truth behind hyperoptimizers' claims about delaying caffeine and cold plunging—and revealing the cognitive biases that make these claims so persuasive—will help you separate signal from noise. This clarity is crucial in evaluating other so-called high-performance methods, protocols, and products, enabling you to avoid unnecessary and sometimes potentially harmful actions.

Not Everyone Is Biologically Wired to Be an Early Bird

We'll begin by challenging step one in the hyperoptimizer playbook for starting your day—the notion that everyone needs to be an early bird.

Biology simply hasn't wired many of us to be that way. Each of us has a *chronotype*—an innate biological predisposition for sleep-wake timing within the twenty-four-hour day.[2,4] If you naturally wake up early, feel most alert in the morning, and wind down in the evening, you're likely a morning chronotype, or early bird. Conversely, if you wake later, reach peak alertness in the evening, and prefer late nights, you're likely a late chronotype, also known as a night owl. The population variation follows a normal distribution, so most people fall somewhere between these extremes.

Imagine gathering a group of people, placing them on the same light-dark schedule, and giving them the freedom to sleep and wake entirely based on their natural inclinations. Over a few days, distinct patterns would emerge: Some individuals would naturally settle into an early bedtime and wake time, while others would gravitate toward staying up and rising later. Additionally, variations in sleep duration would appear, with some needing less sleep and others requiring more. These differences reflect the interplay of biological rhythms, individual sleep needs (the amount of sleep your body requires to function well) and sleep capacity (your ability to obtain sufficient restorative sleep).

Decoding Sleep: How Two Systems Shape Your Alertness and Sleepiness

The *two-process model of sleep regulation* offers an elegant explanation for why we feel sleepy at night and alert during the day and why timing varies between people.[4] The model hinges on two interconnected systems.

The first, the sleep *homeostat* (Process S), functions like an hourglass sand timer, but instead of sand, it tracks the buildup of sleep pressure. This buildup may be marked by the accumulation of a molecule called adenosine in the brain. As the metaphorical timer fills, we feel increasingly sleepy. Sleep acts like flipping the hourglass, clearing away accumulated adenosine and resetting the system for the next day.

The second system involved in sleep regulation is the *circadian pacemaker*, also known as Process C. This is the body's internal clock, located in a small structure in the brain called the suprachiasmatic nucleus—think of it as the "master clock" that keeps time for your body. It spontaneously generates a near twenty-four-hour rhythm regulates when we feel alert and when we feel drowsy.

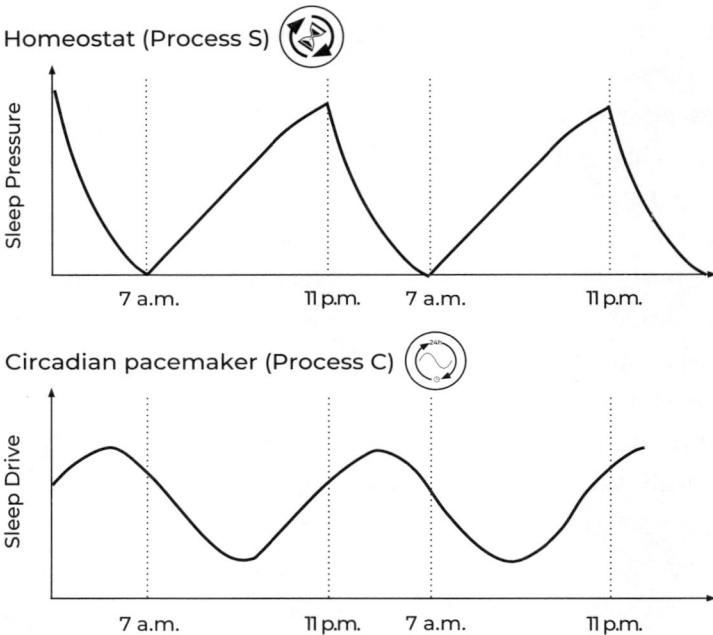

Figure adapted based on Lockley & Foster (2012)

About two to three hours before bedtime Process C peaks—a final push from your circadian system to suppress sleepiness and keep you awake, even as sleep pressure (Process S) builds up from being awake all day—levels of *melatonin*, a hormone often described as the "signal of darkness," also begin to rise. This process, called DLMO (dim light melatonin onset), tells the body that nighttime is approaching and triggers preparations for sleep, though melatonin itself does not directly cause sleep.

Following DLMO, the wake maintenance phase of Process C subsides, the circadian alerting signal diminishes, and sleep pressure peaks. Like a dam finally overflowing, this combination primes the body to fall asleep.

Early birds tend to experience a faster buildup of sleep pressure, prompting them to feel sleepy sooner.[5] Yet this *sleep pressure* dissipates more quickly, allowing them to wake earlier. Night owls, on the other hand, build up sleep pressure more slowly, extending wakefulness into later hours. Early types may also have a slightly faster internal circadian clock, making their day closer to twenty-four hours, while night owls may have a slower clock, nudging their rhythm slightly beyond twenty-four hours.[6]

Imagine two people—an early bird and a night owl—set their alarms for 5:00 a.m. Overnight the early bird's sleep pressure dissipates faster than that of the night owl, so the early bird wakes with less residual *sleep pressure*. Additionally, because of the early bird's faster internal clock, 5:00 a.m. feels like a more natural wake time, while for the night owl, it feels biologically much earlier.

Though both rise at the same time on the clock, the early bird wakes feeling more refreshed and alert, while the night owl wakes at an earlier biological wake time with lingering sleep pressure.[7,8]

How Many People Are Truly Early Birds?

A large-scale Harvard-led study involving 53,689 participants found that roughly 25 percent of people are early birds, another 25 percent are night owls, and the remaining 50 percent fall somewhere in between.[3] Twin and family studies indicate that about half of our chronotype is genetically determined.[2] However, our chronotype changes over time.

Many of us will remember finding it almost impossible to wake up early and wanting to stay up later when we were teenagers. This experience has a biological basis. In addition to needing more sleep (young adults generally need at least eight and a half hours of sleep, with teenagers needing even more), during adolescence, a change in timing between the two systems that control sleep and wakefulness occurs—the homeostat and the circadian pacemaker.

Sleep pressure tends to build up more slowly for older teenagers, and their entrained circadian phase is later, which delays their propensity to sleep until later in the day. This pattern, common to both young men and women, is responsible for teenagers' night owl tendencies, which usually peak between ages fifteen and nineteen. It's not until adulthood, in our early twenties, that sleep and wake times begin to move earlier again. The observation that this change occurs two years earlier for girls than boys suggests that it is driven by underlying biological processes tied to maturation, rather than purely social or environmental factors.

Chronotype changes continue throughout our lifetime, with notable differences between men and women.[3] For example, before age forty, men often tend toward later bedtimes than women, fitting the classic night owl type. But after forty, this flips: On average, women tend to favor later schedules, while men gradually shift to earlier sleep schedules.

For women, sleep timing generally stabilizes between thirty-five and fifty. In contrast, men's sleep preferences continue to drift earlier so that by later adulthood, they generally become earlier chronotypes than women.

Chronotypes can vary by four to six hours between individuals.[3] For instance, an early bird such as Franklin may feel ready to go at 5:00 a.m., but it may take a night owl until 10:00 a.m. to reach the same level of alertness.

Despite the biological basis for chronotype differences, society unfairly continues to maintain biases in favor of early birds. For example, employers tend to perceive early starters as more competent than their later-arriving peers—based solely on arrival time.[9] Research also reveals that supervisors frequently rate later-starting employees as lower performers, even when these employees equal or surpass their early-rising colleagues in both total work hours and objective productivity metrics.[10]

Perhaps it's time to reconsider our veneration of the early start.

The Hidden Health Costs of Living Out of Sync with Your Body Clock

One of the reasons I'm against people promoting the idea that everyone should be an early riser is that encouraging people to shift their sleep schedules and work against their natural chronotype has proven risks and harms.

Daylight saving time, which forces billions to spring forward each year, offers a large-scale natural experiment demonstrating the impact of shifting sleep timing by just one hour.

The spring shift, when the clocks move forward, leads to an average loss of about thirty minutes of sleep per night.[11] Though this may sound minor, it quickly accumulates into a meaningful sleep deficit, leaving many with poorer-quality sleep, lingering morning fatigue, and daytime drowsiness.[12,13]

But the effects extend beyond grogginess. In the days after daylight saving time begins, the risk of heart attacks spikes by 27 percent.[14] Patient safety incidents rise by 18 percent, likely due to clinician fatigue.[15] On the roads, vehicle crashes increase.[16] Circadian misalignment also affects cognitive performance, impairing memory and concentration.[17] Emerging research even suggests that disruptions in sleep timing may alter gut microbiome composition, leading to inflammation and a heightened risk of cardiovascular disease.[18]

In sum, the consequences of even small shifts in sleep timing are far-reaching, affecting everything from mental acuity to heart health. Many of us would benefit from identifying our chronotype and considering how we can align with our natural sleep-wake timing more closely. While achieving a schedule that perfectly matches our biology may be unrealistic, even small changes to make our sleep schedule more consistent and better aligned with our natural tendencies could offer welcome advantages for health and performance.

How to Identify Your Chronotype

Many people already have a sense of their chronotype. If you're still wondering about yours, consider your sleep timing when you're free to go to bed and wake up whenever you want to, such as during a vacation (as long as there are no kids or pets to disturb you). I've met many people who convinced themselves they were early birds because of their work demands, only to reflect on their vacation routines and realize they were more naturally inclined to be night owls.

You could also use a more structured questionnaire tool such as the *Circadian Energy Scale*.[19] The scale includes two questions. Answer each question on a scale from 1 to 5: *1 = Very low, 2 = Low, 3 = Moderate, 4 = High, and 5 = Very high.*

In general, how is your energy level in the *evening*?	
In general, how is your energy level in the *morning*?	
Evening Score – Morning Score =	

You should end up with two numbers: one for your evening energy and the other for your morning energy. When you have these, subtract your morning score from your evening score.

For example, my evening score is 2, and my morning score is 4. Therefore, 2 (evening) – 4 (morning) = -2.

When you have your answer, check it against the following reference ranges to find your type:

> *Morning type: -4 to -2*
> *Intermediate type: -1 to 1*
> *Evening type: 2 to 4*

You can see that with a score of -2, I fall just into the morning-type category.

Other academically validated surveys and methods offer more accurate, precise insights and a detailed understanding of your biological rhythms. However, the results of the Circadian Energy Scale are reasonably consistent with more extensive, validated survey instruments, providing a quick, low-effort method for estimating chronotype.[19]

Whatever method you choose, once you have a sense of your chronotype, you can begin adjusting your daily rhythm—such as scheduling your wake time to better coincide with your chronotype and natural tendency.

Can You Change Your Chronotype?

Many people are curious about whether they can overcome their biological propensity and change their chronotype to become more of an early bird, for example.

We can change our sleep and wake timing—traveling and adapting to a new time zone makes this obvious. Provided you're sleeping adequately, you can adjust your environment and behavior in your current location. However, this does not represent a true change to our underlying chronotype or need for sleep, both of which have strong genetic components.[2,20] Any modifications typically require consistent effort and are unlikely to become permanent without ongoing intervention.

Rather than trying to change our chronotype, most of us would benefit more from stabilizing our circadian rhythm by going to sleep and waking up at consistent times aligned with our natural tendencies. This approach would likely improve our sleep and make it easier to wake up feeling alert and ready to tackle the day ahead.[6,21,22]

Should We Stop Hitting Snooze?

Let's take a quick look back at the hyperoptimizer playbook. After setting your alarm for 5:00 a.m.—or earlier (chronotype be damned)—the next mandate is to avoid hitting snooze at all costs. But is it truly one of the cardinal sins of self-improvement?

A study from the University of Notre Dame explored which traits are linked to hitting the snooze button.[23] Among the 57 percent of participants who reported snoozing, several characteristics stood out: They were more likely to be younger, have later chronotypes, experience more disturbed sleep, and be less conscientious (the personality trait of being responsible, careful, or diligent).

It would be easy to jump on the final point and claim that laziness causes snoozing. However, it's important to note that the findings of this study were associative. It's equally likely that the tendency to snooze reflects biological and social factors associated with being young. As noted earlier, teenagers and young adults often have later chronotypes. Societal expectations for early starts (work, school) can clash with their internal rhythms, leading them to snooze to cope with an imposed wake time that doesn't match their biology. Additionally, the prefrontal cortex, a brain region responsible for self-regulation and impulse control, is still developing in younger people, potentially making it more challenging to adhere to a consistent sleep schedule.[24]

* * *

The self-help saints and hyperoptimizers often suggest that snoozing your alarm may negatively affect the biological processes that govern sleep. But is this true?

A study including researchers from the prestigious Karolinska Institute—one of the world's foremost medical universities—revealed that snoozing did not appear to affect the cortisol awakening response—a spike in cortisol levels driven by the circadian clock that helps prepare the body for the day ahead—suggesting that snoozing doesn't necessarily undermine your body's natural wake-up process.[25] In fact, the researchers highlighted some benefits associated with a brief snooze. For example, among people with later chronotypes and those who felt particularly sleepy upon waking, snoozing helped alleviate sleep inertia—the grogginess and impaired alertness we sometimes feel right after waking up.

So, what does this mean? In an ideal world, we wouldn't need to hit snooze because we'd get all the sleep our bodies require without needing an alarm to wake us. It's also clear that we would benefit from maintaining consistent sleep and wake times. Nonetheless, a recent consensus statement from the world's leading sleep scientists takes a pragmatic and evidence-based view. While they highlight the benefits of consistency in sleep timing, they note that getting an extra one or two hours of sleep on weekends, if needed, can reduce some of the health risks associated with shorter sleep during the workweek.[26]

As always, more research is required, but these findings should encourage us not to be hard on ourselves or others if we choose to grab some extra sleep. With that said, if you feel you would benefit from more sleep, it's better to set your alarm for as late as possible and sleep uninterrupted until it goes off, rather than waking up and hitting snooze. This approach maximizes both the duration and quality of your sleep.

Many people enjoy waking up early and find it beneficial, which may align perfectly with their body clock. However, the self-improvement world's obsession with early rising and the avoidance of sleeping relatively later is more likely a misinterpretation of evidence—or a manifestation of *puritanical bias,* the tendency to reduce complex issues to personal shortcomings while dismissing other factors—than a position grounded in strong empirical evidence.[27]

Should We Prioritize Sunlight in the Morning?

Despite our differences, I share the hyperoptimizers' recognition of light's importance. No one's circadian rhythm aligns perfectly with a twenty-four-hour day, so we need daily cues to stay in sync with the earth's cycle. Light is the most powerful *zeitgeber*—which literally means time giver or time cue—for our circadian clock. This need for alignment and the importance of the timing of light-dark cycles was highlighted in groundbreaking 1960s experiments conducted by French researcher Michel Siffre.[28]

Siffre spent 179 days isolated in a cave in the French Alps, free from natural light or timekeeping devices, to observe his body's natural sleep-wake patterns. Without any external cues, his internal clock stretched to a twenty-four-and-a-half-hour day, and his sleep-wake cycle varied wildly, sometimes lasting forty or even fifty hours. When he resurfaced, Siffre's sense of time had drifted a full month behind reality.

Siffre's work and subsequent research dispelled the notion that our circadian rhythms are exactly twenty-four hours, showing instead that we rely on environmental signals, the strongest of which is light, to stay aligned.[4,29]

These findings also suggest that overoptimizers may overstate the emphasis on morning light if the goal is simply to regulate, rather than shift, your circadian rhythm. For instance, while morning light is effective for phase-advancing the circadian clock (shifting it earlier), this could be counterproductive for those who naturally lean toward morningness. As a general principle, maintaining consistent sleep-wake patterns, with appropriate light exposure during the day, is more critical for overall circadian health than focusing so much on morning light exposure.

Prioritizing bright light exposure during the day is essential for maintaining a healthy circadian rhythm. Natural daylight is the best option, even if the sky is overcast. If stepping outside isn't feasible, bright indoor light can also help, provided it meets the threshold of sufficient melanopic equivalent daylight illuminance (melEDI).

MelEDI lux is a measure of light intensity that reflects its effect on the human circadian system, particularly the pathways in the brain that regulate sleep, alertness, and biological rhythms.[29] Evidence indicates that for most of the day, we should aim to be in environments with at least 250 melanopic equivalent daylight illuminance (melEDI) lux on the vertical plane at eye level. To make this more tangible, 250 melEDI lux is comparable to sitting in a room near a window, even on a cloudy day. However, note that you will likely need to face the window; otherwise, the light reaching your eyes may not meet this threshold.

By contrast, dim lights to 10 melEDI lux or lower in the three hours leading up to sleep. This intensity is comparable to the light from a small lamp in the corner of a room. During sleep, your bedroom should not exceed 1 lux.

In addition to sleep and wakefulness, light and circadian rhythm synchronization also influences our metabolism and psychology.[4,30] For example, circadian rhythm disruptions are associated with a twofold increased risk of metabolic syndrome and diabetes/prediabetes.[31] Light exposure has an antidepressant effect, and bright, blue-enriched light—similar to a sunny day outdoors—can significantly boost mood.[4,30] Natural daylight exposure also improves sleep quality and can extend sleep duration.[4,30] So, rather than fixating on morning light alone, focus first on establishing regular sleep and wake times, coupled with adequate light exposure during your active hours and darkness during your sleep period.[26,29]

Do We Really Need to Delay Our Morning Coffee?

As we work through the hyperoptimizers' guide for starting the day, we find step four and the increasingly popular claim that we should delay caffeine intake for one and a half to two hours after waking. This instruction is often accompanied by convincing-sounding neuroscientific arguments and the suggestion that it will help you avoid an afternoon crash—the sense that we have a dip in energy in the afternoon.

Perhaps you're unfamiliar with the idea of delaying your morning caffeine intake, but as I mentioned earlier, this practice provides a striking example of how hyperoptimizers leverage cognitive biases to shape our thinking—often in misleading ways. The so-called delay-caffeine protocol has gained enough traction that a team of twenty researchers, led by the esteemed Professor Jose Antonio, a prominent expert in nutrition, health, and human performance, recently conducted a comprehensive review to investigate whether evidence supports the claims behind it.[32]

After scouring the academic literature, the researchers concluded that "a fundamental basis for suggesting that delaying caffeine intake in the early waking hours would prevent an afternoon 'crash' is completely lacking."

To cut a long story short, the scientific-sounding explanation proposed by the delay-caffeine advocates is incorrect.

Remember adenosine—the chemical signaler that builds up throughout the day, creating *sleep pressure* like an hourglass timer filling with sand, before dissipating during sleep? It's generally accepted that caffeine works its magic by blocking adenosine receptors, enhancing alertness and cognitive sharpness—especially if you're running on less sleep.[33]

Proponents of delaying caffeine suggest that adenosine levels continue to dissipate even after waking. Their logic is that consuming caffeine too soon blocks adenosine receptors before adenosine has fully dissipated, so adenosine molecules linger, waiting to cause the afternoon crash after the caffeine has worn off. According to this theory, delaying caffeine for 90 to 120 minutes allows adenosine to dissipate without interference.

Beware of Biological Plausibility Bias

The adenosine theory above sounds intuitive, but it's an example of *biological plausibility bias*—we're inclined to believe something without looking deeper when an explanation sounds logical. In fact, the hyperoptimizers' explanation is *entirely contrary to the scientific evidence.*

Adenosine does not continue to dissipate after we wake up. Rather, the opposite happens. There is a rapid increase in adenosine after waking— imagine the hourglass sand timer being flipped as soon as we wake up—so delaying caffeine on this basis does not make any sense.[34, 35, 36]

Supporters of the delay protocol offer another argument: They claim that consuming caffeine immediately after waking prolongs the spike in cortisol (the stress hormone) that occurs naturally based on circadian time. This also sounds plausible; no one wants to interfere with natural hormone cycles. But once again, there's no evidence that caffeine disrupts the normal pattern of cortisol release throughout the day, making this argument equally unfounded.[37]

In summary, both claims—about adenosine clearance and cortisol— are unsupported by scientific evidence. This hasn't stopped people from promoting caffeine delay all over the internet, though.

Rather than delaying caffeine, consuming it immediately after waking may actually be beneficial in some cases. For example, if you start the day with exercise or physical tasks, caffeine can enhance endurance and strength, making physical effort feel less demanding.[38]

If you enjoy a morning coffee, there's no real reason to delay it, no matter how often hyperoptimizers repeat this *zombie claim*—an idea that just will not die.

Instead of obsessing over unnecessary protocols, we might benefit more from reflecting on the well-documented health benefits of coffee consumption. For example, drinking two to three cups of ground coffee daily is associated with a 27 percent reduction in all-cause mortality—the risk of dying from anything during a given period.[39] Decaf and instant coffee drinkers also experienced reduced risk, with drops of 14 percent and 11 percent, respectively.[39] Further, a large-scale review found regular coffee consumption was associated with an 18 percent reduced cancer risk and lower risks of several neurological, metabolic, and liver conditions.[40]

Of course, coffee and caffeine may be unsuitable for certain health conditions, so it's wise to consult a medical professional if you have concerns. As noted earlier, we should also be mindful of caffeine's impact on sleep— we'll cover this in chapter 4—but overall, your morning coffee likely brings more benefits than downsides.

Should You Start the Day with a Cold Plunge?

We've reached step five in the *hyperoptimizer playbook* for starting your day: replace coffee with a cold plunge.

Interest in deliberate cold exposure and cold-water immersion is soaring. The value of the cold plunge tub market is expected to reach a value of nearly $500 million in the coming years.[41] According to reports from organizers of executive retreats and team-building events, more than 50 percent of clients request cold immersion experiences.[41]

But is it all that its adherents claim? Let's take a look.

1. COLD EXPOSURE MAY BOOST METABOLISM, BUT IT MAKES US EAT MORE

One of the most popular claims about cold exposure is that it boosts metabolism. Some basis for this exists. For example, studies have shown a twofold increase in metabolic rate during cold exposure.[42] But ice bath advocates often omit a key detail: This study was conducted on *mice*. Additionally, the same research found that the mice ate more when exposed to cold, offsetting any calorie burn from the increased metabolic rate and ultimately preventing weight loss.[42] A similar effect seems to occur in humans: Cold exposure lowers leptin, a hormone that helps regulate appetite, often leading to increased food intake.[43]

2. COLD EXPOSURE MAY "BURN FAT," BUT THE PRACTICAL IMPACT IS IRRELEVANT

Most research on the metabolic effects of cold exposure has been conducted on animals. While some findings might be relevant to humans, critical differences weaken many of the bold claims of cold exposure proponents. For instance, compared with other mammals, humans have very little brown fat—a type of fat activated by cold exposure to generate heat.[44] So while brown fat activation may technically increase metabolism—a common claim that *hyperoptimizers* use to support their arguments and professed benefits—its practical effect on humans is inconsequential.[45]

3. COLD EXPOSURE ADVOCATES ARE VULNERABLE TO CONFIRMATION BIAS

Some of the hyperoptimizers' favorite cold-water immersion studies also lack rigor—the studies were not conducted with enough thoroughness or precision. A recent example involves a widely promoted study that claimed cold exposure significantly reduced abdominal fat in soldiers.[46] These findings went viral, but a closer look at the study raised serious issues. For one, it was small, and the results barely met statistical significance, suggesting they might have been due to chance. Additionally, the study's analytical methods were questionable, sparking concern among scientists. The journal ultimately retracted the study, deeming its analyses unreliable.

The retraction never made it to the social media feeds of those who had enthusiastically promoted the study—proof, perhaps, that cold exposure doesn't chill *confirmation bias:* the human tendency to highlight information that aligns with our beliefs while ignoring anything that challenges them.

If your goal is metabolic health, prioritizing adequate sleep and regular exercise, as discussed in later chapters, is far more effective than an icy plunge.[47,48]

4. MANY COLD EXPOSURE CLAIMS LEVERAGE MULTIPLE COGNITIVE BIASES

Another popular hyperoptimizer claim is that "cold plunging increases dopamine by 250 percent," which "boosts mood, motivation, and cognitive performance." However, this claim is a textbook example of how influencers leverage cognitive biases to gain trust, avoid scrutiny, and encourage us that we should be *hyperoptimizers,* too.

Cognitive biases used to persuade and sometimes mislead include the following:

> **Precision Bias: Use a Very Specific Number**
> The first step in the *hyperoptimizers' guide to persuasion* is to state a very specific number with great confidence. In this case, saying "a 250 percent increase" rather than simply "an increase" leverages *precision bias*—we tend to assume that very specific figures reflect careful measurement, reliable research, and accuracy. Precision also lends an air of authority, obscuring uncertainties, limitations, or errors in data collection and analysis. As a result we're inclined to accept claims without looking further.
>
> **Biological Plausibility Bias: Offer a Logical-Sounding Argument**
> Next, as with the delay-caffeine myth, you must propose a logical-sounding biological mechanism to support your claim. In this example, the claim that cold plunging boosts mood, motivation, and cognitive performance is based on the following (flawed) logic:
>
> Cold plunging raises dopamine levels.
>
> Dopamine in the brain is linked to mood, motivation, and cognitive performance.
>
> Therefore, cold plunging must improve mood, motivation, and cognitive performance.
>
> *Biological plausibility bias* leads us to assume that the claim is true and that there is a cause-and-effect relationship without digging

deeper, simply because there is a logical-sounding biological link that seems like it should be true.

Use SANE (Seductive Allure of Neuroscience Explanations)
The pièce de résistance in the hyperoptimizers' guide is SANE—the *seductive allure of neuroscience explanations*—a term coined after research revealed that we are more likely to identify bad explanations as good when they contain neuroscience information.[49]

They also observed that explanations are more satisfying if they contain neuroscientific terms and imagery, even if they are irrelevant. In this cold plunging example, the liberal references to *dopamine*—which many people recognize as a neurotransmitter—could trigger SANE. Many social media posts layer on (irrelevant) brain scan images to enhance the effect.

This combination of biases has helped propel the claim that cold plunging boosts brain dopamine, with all its proposed benefits, all over the internet. However, if we recognize these biases and pause to examine the evidence more thoroughly, we'll find a whole other story.

The Truth About Cold Plunges and Dopamine

The misunderstanding began because the people making the cold plunge claims didn't either read or accurately interpret the original research that reported the "250 percent" finding. The 250 percent figure actually refers to an increase in *plasma dopamine* in the body, *not* an increase in *brain dopamine*.[50] This is a critical error because dopamine plays different roles in the body relative to the brain.

In the brain, dopamine is a *neurotransmitter* that influences motivation, mood, movement, and cognition. However, in the body—where dopamine was measured in the oft-quoted cold plunge study—dopamine primarily acts as a hormone, driving physiological responses such as increased urine production and shivering. But precision bias tends to minimize scrutiny, so the distinction between dopamine in the brain and the body is often overlooked.

Rather than speculating about cognitive benefits, a more accurate interpretation of the study's findings would note that the 250 percent increase in plasma dopamine was associated with a 163 percent increase in urine output, but that doesn't make for a social media–friendly headline.

It's also important to note that while cold-water immersion *may* raise brain dopamine levels, to date, this has never been measured directly. For otherwise healthy individuals, it remains unclear whether intentionally and significantly elevating dopamine beyond the brain's tightly regulated levels is either achievable or beneficial.[51] Nonetheless, *biological plausibility bias* leads us to accept the seemingly logical explanation of the mechanisms and benefits of boosting brain dopamine without considering alternatives.

Hyperoptimizer anecdotes also abound about how the dopamine boost from cold plunging increases focus, clarity, and mental acuity. SANE makes this claim sound convincing. However, this bias inclines us to discount other evidence, such as the comprehensive review of research that found that cold exposure impairs cognitive performance during and immediately after exposure rather than enhancing it.[52]

The hyperoptimizers' explanations also neglect that other types of physical or psychological stress activate the brain's dopamine circuits, triggering immediate changes in neural function.[53] Any proposed benefits are far from unique. As we'll explore in chapters 4 and 5, if you're seeking ways to improve mood, enhance alertness, and boost cognitive function, prioritizing quality sleep and regular exercise are proven, effective, and likely safer alternatives to an ice bath.

Morning Exercise Likely Offers Greater Benefits than Cold Exposure

Specifically in the context of boosting alertness in the morning, exercise, in particular, can be very effective. A short morning aerobic exercise session, such as a fifty-minute moderate-intensity run or cycle, where you're breathing faster but not out of breath, can also boost mood and cognitive performance for several hours.[54,55]

Overall, the evidence for cold-water exposure and its benefits is far weaker than it's made out to be, but we shouldn't feel bad about being drawn in by hyperoptimizers' convincing explanations. All humans are vulnerable to cognitive biases, and many influencers appear to give us good reasons—such as being highly credentialed—to believe them. But next time you hear convincing-sounding claims from a self-improvement influencer about cold plunging, or any of their regimes or methods for that matter, ask yourself whether they might be leveraging cognitive biases to encourage unthinking acceptance.

Don't Overlook the Safety Risks of Cold-Water Immersion

It would be remiss of me not to address the safety risks associated with cold-water immersion, regardless of time of day. Professor Mike Tipton—considered one of the world's foremost experts on this topic—coauthored a paper with the telling title *Cold Water Immersion: Kill or Cure?*[56] The authors emphasize that cold-water immersion is a significant cause of worldwide fatalities. Physiological responses such as *cold shock*, *autonomic conflict*, and *physical incapacitation* can lead to drowning or cardiac arrest, even after brief exposure under seemingly controlled conditions. Additionally, cold-water immersion is linked to a high incidence of irregular heart rhythms, even among healthy individuals.[57]

The evidence supporting the benefits of cold-water exposure is relatively thin compared with the well-documented risks. Most studies are small, often limited to a single gender, and vary widely in methodology. Many rely on subjective claims or anecdotal reports rather than rigorous data. And despite what influencers suggest, no established optimal dose of cold exposure exists.[56]

I'm not denying that people have experienced benefits from cold-water immersion. I spent several years working for a Finnish company and have fond memories of jumping into ice holes with friends and colleagues (ideally followed by a sauna).

However, it's possible that many of these benefits stem from the placebo effect, as we anticipate positive outcomes. Additionally, aspects unrelated to cold exposure—such as time spent outdoors with friends—could play a significant role.

The possibility that placebo or other factors contribute to its benefits shouldn't diminish the value of the experience. However, the thorough, balanced research of Professor Tipton and his colleagues highlights the need for caution. Before deliberate cold exposure and cold-water immersion are widely promoted as routine practices—whether first thing in the morning or later in the day—additional research and a careful assessment of risks are essential.

Is Breakfast Really the Most Important Meal of the Day?

So perhaps the cold plunge isn't for everyone—but should we approach breakfast with the same skepticism? While hyperoptimizers preach the first five steps of their morning routine with unshakable conviction, they appear surprisingly unsure about the day's first meal.

Some will tell you that breakfast is essential. Others will recommend skipping it, particularly if they are fans of *intermittent fasting* (a topic we will address in chapter 6). Many people suggest that breakfast benefits health, cognition, and performance, but overall, the evidence is mixed, revealing a nuanced picture rather than a clear mandate.

> **Metabolic Rate and Physical Activity:** Breakfast doesn't appear to influence metabolic rate, though skipping it may lead to reduced daily physical activity.[58]

> **Hunger and Satiety:** A high-protein breakfast can help curb hunger later in the day, but this effect is strongest after a good night's sleep—a link we'll explore in upcoming chapters.[59]

> **Weight Loss and Caloric Intake:** In a randomized controlled trial among adults aiming to lose weight, skipping breakfast had no discernable effect on weight loss.[60] Similarly, a randomized controlled trial focusing on overweight and obese women found that breakfast intake did not significantly affect lunchtime calories or total daily calorie intake.[61]

> **Cognitive Performance:** People tend to concentrate better after eating a high-protein, low-carb breakfast compared with skipping it.[61] However, the impact on cognition isn't always consistent: Among adolescents and children, including in a clinical trial, breakfast didn't significantly affect cognitive performance.[62,63]

Nutrient Intake: Skipping breakfast increases the risk that children and young people may miss out on essential nutrients, such as vitamins.[64]

Physical Performance: The effects of breakfast on physical performance are clearer. Skipping breakfast can impair resistance exercise performance, especially in those who typically eat breakfast.[65] Interestingly, one study found that simply believing we have had breakfast—via a taste- and texture-matched placebo—was enough to improve endurance.[66]

In summary, breakfast may support physical performance, nutrient intake, and concentration for some people, but it isn't a magic bullet for metabolism or weight loss. The potential benefits of breakfast are nuanced, influenced by factors such as sleep quality, exercise habits, and individual lifestyle. The mixed findings also highlight the challenges of conducting and interpreting nutrition research—a topic we will tackle in chapter 6.

The answer to whether breakfast is the most important meal of the day depends on who you are and what you are trying to achieve.

Be Your Own Scientist All Day Long

Arguably, the most crucial element of starting your day is finding an approach that genuinely works for you. As we conclude this first chapter, let's introduce a practical tool—*expected value calculations*—that can help you experiment with your morning routine and other strategies in this book.

Drawn from probability theory and decision-making frameworks commonly used in economics, finance, and game theory, *expected value calculations* provide a method for estimating the potential outcomes of our choices and actions. If an action looks like it will consistently offer more benefits than downsides across various scenarios, it has a positive expected value and could be worth pursuing. Conversely, if the drawbacks outweigh the benefits, it holds a negative expected value and may be best avoided.

Using this framework can empower you to make decisions grounded in long-term benefit, enabling you to tailor a routine that aligns with your goals and truly enhances your day.

You can calculate *expected value* as follows:

Expected Value = (Potential Benefits × Probability of Benefits) -
(Potential Risks × Probability of Risks) - Implementation Costs

For example, in the context of morning cold-water immersion, I would argue that the well-documented potential risks outweigh the uncertain benefits.[56] Adding in the cost in time and money puts the nail in the coffin. Here's how I came to that conclusion based on my personal context using the *expected value formula*:

Potential Benefits: 4/10 (reflecting the lack of strong academic evidence)

Probability of Benefits: 0.5 (50 percent chance of realizing meaningful benefits, based on weak evidence and lack of research in humans)

Potential Risks: 6/10 (reflecting the potential severity of adverse reactions)

Probability of Risks: 0.3 (30 percent chance, based on the potential for adverse reactions, even in otherwise healthy people)

Implementation Costs: 5/10 (equipment cost: 2/10 + opportunity cost in time: 3/10)

Therefore,

*My Expected Value = (4 × 0.5) - (6 × 0.3) - 5 = 2 - 1.8 - 5 = -***4.8**

By contrast, using the time I would have spent in an ice bath for a brisk morning walk—combining exercise and natural light exposure—likely offers significantly better risk-adjusted benefits.

Achieving Morning Mastery

However you start your day, give yourself some grace. Avoid comparisons with others who may have entirely different biological rhythms or personal circumstances. Even if you thrive on structure, there's a strong case for holding your routine lightly. Few morning routines survive their first contact with Monday. As a general principle, aim for simplicity over sophistication and consistency over complexity.

Rather than setting us up for success, overly rigid routines may make us vulnerable to life's inevitable curveballs. Instead of aiming for unshakable self-discipline and defined dopamine percentages, we could benefit from embracing shoshin—the beginner's mind.

True morning mastery might not be about achieving the perfect start but rather developing the resilience to roll with the punches and the openness and curiosity to learn from whatever comes our way.

CHAPTER 1 REVIEW

In this chapter we explored the self-improvement world's obsession with morning routines and discovered why there's no universal right way to start our days. We examined common morning practices promoted by *hyperoptimizers* and found that many lack scientific support. We then uncovered evidence-based approaches for developing routines that align with our individual biology.

KEY INSIGHTS

CHRONOTYPE DETERMINES OUR OPTIMAL SCHEDULE

- Approximately 25 percent of us are early birds, 25 percent are night owls, and 50 percent fall somewhere in between.
- Our chronotype is roughly 50 percent genetically determined.
- When we fight our natural chronotype, we risk health, safety, and performance issues.

MORNING CAFFEINE DELAY IS A MYTH

- Delaying morning caffeine has no scientific basis (it relies on biological plausibility bias).
- Claims about adenosine clearance and cortisol disruption are unsupported.
- Regular coffee consumption is associated with various health benefits.

COLD EXPOSURE CLAIMS NEED SCRUTINY

- Cold exposure benefits are often overstated.
- The "250 percent dopamine increase" claim misinterprets research.
- Cold exposure carries significant safety risks that are often overlooked.

LIGHT EXPOSURE REGULATES OUR RHYTHM

- Consistent light-dark cycles help regulate our circadian rhythm.
- During the day, aim to be in environments with at least 250 melEDI lux on the vertical plane at eye level.

- Dim lights to 10 melEDI lux or lower in the three hours leading up to sleep.

PRACTICAL ACTIONS

1. IDENTIFY YOUR CHRONOTYPE

- Take the two-question Circadian Energy Scale assessment.
- Observe your natural sleep patterns during free days.
- Consider how your energy levels vary throughout your day.

2. ASSESS YOUR ALIGNMENT WITH YOUR CHRONOTYPE

- Do you wake up feeling refreshed or force yourself awake with an alarm every day?
- Could you adjust your morning schedule to better align with your chronotype?
- What could you do to make your sleep-wake timing more consistent?

3. CALCULATE YOUR EXPECTED VALUE

- Use this framework to evaluate changes or plans you're considering.
- Consider the potential benefits and the probability of experiencing them.
- Weigh against potential risks and their probability.
- Factor in implementation costs.

Remember This

Rather than copying trending morning routines, focus on aligning your mornings with your natural chronotype and energy patterns. The most effective routine is one you can maintain consistently.

Looking Ahead

In our next chapter, we'll explore how to structure our workdays to find a new rhythm of effort and recovery.

CHAPTER 2

REGENERATIVE WORKDAYS: FIND A NEW RHYTHM OF EFFORT AND RECOVERY

Why does it feel like we're working longer but have less time than ever?

Something about work isn't working.

I've had the privilege of researching, advising, and speaking with organizations in over thirty-five countries—from Formula One teams and Fortune 500 giants to fledgling start-ups and small nonprofits. Despite their vast differences, the *knowledge workers*—the people driving value through cognitive rather than physical tasks—often share common goals: They want to feel *efficient*, *effective*, *decisive*, *focused*, *energized*, and *well rested*.

Yet for many, this experience remains elusive.

Chances are, you can relate.

More Meetings, Less Meaningful Work

Calendars are overloaded—the volume of weekly meetings has increased by 153 percent in recent years.[67] Yet these meetings rarely make efficient use of time. Many knowledge workers doubt they even need to attend a third of the meetings they're invited to.[68] When they do turn up, 92 percent admit to multitasking—a desperate attempt to chip away at an endless to-do list.[69]

Outside meetings, the pressure to appear to be working fuels *productivity theater*: 54 percent of knowledge workers feel compelled to signal their digital presence at specific times, creating the illusion of continual engagement if they're not working constructively.[70] On average, employees spend an extra sixty-seven minutes online each day, such as by sending low-priority emails or "liking" chat messages, just to reassure colleagues they're still on the clock.[70]

Chasing Focus in a World of Distraction

Ideally, knowledge workers say they would have four uninterrupted hours each day to focus.[71] In reality, they spend 10 percent of their time toggling between applications, with interruptions striking every eleven minutes.[72,73] *Digital debt* is mounting, with emails and notifications arriving faster than they can be processed. A total of 84 percent keep their inboxes open at all times, and 70 percent read emails within six seconds of arrival.[74] The need to stay connected even extends to the bathroom, where 42 percent admit to replying to messages.[75] This constant connectivity and task-switching take a toll: Refocusing after each interruption can take up to twenty-three minutes, with the cost of fragmented attention and communication overload totaling an estimated 180 hours lost annually per employee.[76] Consequently, despite a 13 percent rise in working hours, 64 percent still feel there's never enough time to get everything done.[67,73]

Running on Empty

A side effect of the increase in meetings is that the number of overlapping invitations has grown by 46 percent.[67] Many knowledge workers find that their meetings are booked back-to-back. As a result half of employees rarely, if ever, get to take breaks during the workday.[71]

Unsurprisingly, 22 percent of employees in the average organization now show signs of burnout.[77] Rather than feeling efficient, focused, and energized, many knowledge workers are overwhelmed, distracted, and drained.

The Badge of Busy: When Relentless Work Becomes a Professional Identity

Responses to this challenge are polarized. At one extreme we find knowledge workers who have embraced *hustle culture*. *Hustlers* are to the workplace what hyperoptimizers are to morning routines. Rather than hiding or minimizing the brutal demands of always-on work—late nights, missed family dinners, and constant travel—advocates of *hustle culture* wear these sacrifices as badges of honor, amplifying and even celebrating the grinding aspects of their work.[78] As one consultant put it, discussing long hours and sky-high air-miles accounts becomes "a sort of indication for how tough your job is"—a perverse form of professional bragging rights.[78]

This isn't simple masochism, though. Rather, it's a coping strategy—what could be seen as exploitation is transformed into professional currency. The aspects that friends and family view as problematic—3:00 a.m. emails, canceled social plans, and constant availability—prove exceptional commitment and value to clients and customers.

However, this embrace of extreme work isn't without its contradictions, particularly between what is said in public and what is expressed in private. My academic research examines the relationship between well-being and performance in some of the world's most demanding workplaces.[79] The same consultants who boasted about their punishing schedules to clients and colleagues would often criticize these practices and express their concerns about burnout when we spoke in confidence.

The Quiet Quitters: Doing Less Speaks Volumes

At the other end of the spectrum, in stark contrast to *hustle culture*, we find a growing movement of knowledge workers embracing *quiet quitting*—a deliberate decision to do only what the job requires and nothing more. Research suggests that up to 50 percent of the workforce is drawn to this approach.[80]

Quiet quitting might sound like disengagement rebranded, but it's more nuanced. As we'll explore in chapter 7, *quiet quitting* may stem from a mindset—overestimating the harm associated with stress and underestimating one's ability to cope. However, it may also signal a breakdown in the psychological contract between employer and employee.

Younger employees, in particular, report significant declines in feeling supported at work and in seeing opportunities for growth.[81] Employees respond by pulling back their discretionary efforts when companies fail to deliver on work-life balance and professional development promises.

Unsurprisingly, *quiet quitting* appears to be most prevalent in knowledge work settings, where the boundaries between work and life have become increasingly blurred. In this light *quiet quitting* might better be understood not as withdrawal but as an overcorrection in response to always-on work.

Our Approach to Knowledge Work Needs a Reboot

You may not see yourself fitting neatly into either *hustle culture* or *quiet quitting,* but many knowledge workers oscillate somewhere between the two. They might spend weeks—or even months—feeling highly engaged, putting in long hours, and keeping pace with demanding workloads. But eventually, the toll sets in: They become overloaded, exhausted, and apathetic.

After a relatively brief disengagement period (quiet quitting) convinced that extra effort isn't worth it, a new project comes along, and they dive right back in, beginning the cycle all over again.

We can't lay the responsibility for this problem or its solution entirely at the employees' feet. Organizations and leaders play a crucial role in creating work environments that enable employees to meet their responsibilities without sacrificing their well-being—often requiring structural and cultural shifts. However, employees can take steps to break the cycle of overwork and disengagement by finding a *third way* characterized by new rhythms of more efficient work, enhanced focus, and effective rest.

Applying Lessons from Endurance Sport to the Workplace

Long before I turned my focus to the performance of knowledge workers, I spent several years in the South of France, chasing my dream of becoming a professional cyclist. I wasn't the most naturally gifted athlete, but I believed I could make up for it by outworking everyone else: riding further, training longer, and pushing harder.

At first this approach seemed to pay off. But soon I found myself exhausted, overtrained, and stuck in a cycle of diminishing returns. I'd push myself relentlessly for a few weeks until my body demanded a break. Then I'd spend days in a fog of exhaustion, barely accomplishing anything on or off the bike, until I could summon the energy to start the cycle again.

Thankfully, I realized this strategy was flawed. I found a new coach who taught me to focus on the *quality,* not just the *quantity,* of my training.

Together, we structured my sessions around the right mix of frequency, intensity, and duration to maximize improvement. He also taught me the value of proactive recovery—learning to rest and recharge before I hit the wall so I could sustain my performance rather than crashing and needing weeks to recover. The new approach was effective, and I had the opportunity to race full-time for several years.

My cycling career ultimately didn't reach the heights I'd hoped for. I'd explored my physical limits but realized I wasn't destined for athletic greatness. Still, the experience sparked a lifelong passion for human performance. Back in the UK, after finishing my undergraduate degree, like many former athletes, I launched my own coaching business.

Road cycling was on its way to becoming the new golf, and I found my core client base among knowledge workers. They were a motley crew of management consultants, technology workers, and finance professionals—many on the *hustle culture* side of the equation—who worked eighty or more hours a week and wanted to race for 180 kilometers on the weekend.

Initially, I focused solely on their physical training. However, it quickly became clear that their demanding work schedules couldn't be ignored when designing their programs. I set out to learn everything I could about knowledge work and soon recognized a familiar pattern.

Too Many Knowledge Workers Focus on Quantity over Quality

Most of my clients were caught up in a cycle of *quantity* over *quality*. They spent long hours at their laptops, constantly switching between tasks and juggling competing demands, without pausing to think about how to work efficiently and effectively. Breaks were rare and usually taken out of sheer exhaustion. Their main performance benchmark was hours worked without considering their natural rhythms of energy and focus.

Week by week their routines mirrored my early training days in France: intense bouts of effort until they hit a wall, followed by unproductive days marred by guilt, only to plunge back into overwork.

Observing this cycle sparked an idea: Could I apply principles from physical endurance training to develop a more sustainable approach to knowledge work performance?

The highly quantifiable nature of cycling has always appealed to me.

As I alluded to earlier, I began to see real improvements when I started to pay attention to *how* I was training rather than mindlessly accumulating more hours. Understanding my training zones—specific intensity ranges that help athletes structure their workouts—was crucial. These zones provided the basis to work smarter, not just harder, by precisely dosing my effort to get the most out of my training time without burning out.

While training zones can be divided more finely, we can reduce most models to three levels, such as the following:

Zone one (**low intensity**)—the easiest level of training. You're working out, but you can still easily hold a conversation.

Zone two (**moderate intensity**)—a challenging but not necessarily effective no-man's-land.*

Zone three (**high intensity**)—the hardest level. You're working very hard, you're breathing heavily, and your muscles feel like they are really burning.

Above zone three are very short sprint efforts, which may only last a few seconds.

Contrary to popular belief, elite endurance athletes don't spend most of their time pushing hard in zone three. World-class cross-country skiers, for instance, dedicate about 80 percent of their annual five hundred training hours to low-intensity zone one.[82] Only 10 to 20 percent is reserved for high-intensity efforts. This *polarized* approach—favoring either low or high intensity, with relatively less time at moderate intensity—has consistently proven more effective for improving key endurance markers than a heavy focus on moderate or high intensities.[83]

---

* Zone two is not to be confused with zone two training, which is often discussed in fitness and health circles and based on a five-zone system. We'll cover this in more detail in chapter 5, which focuses on *regenerative fitness.*

Knowledge Work Is a Cognitive Endurance Activity

My idea was to approach knowledge work as a *cognitive endurance activity* using an intensity-zone-based polarized model. The goal was to encourage knowledge workers to look beyond hours as a proxy for productivity and focus instead on how they were working. By 2015 this concept had taken shape as a framework I called *Cognitive Gears*.[84]

When I first developed *Cognitive Gears,* it was simply a heuristic—a rule of thumb. However, recent research has provided a neuroscientific basis, focusing on the locus coeruleus—a tiny, blue-tinged cluster of neurons in the brainstem.[85,86]

The locus coeruleus is the brain's main source of noradrenaline—a neurotransmitter that plays a key role in our level of alertness. When a cell in the locus coeruleus activates, it releases noradrenaline along its pathways to other neurons, increasing their sensitivity to incoming signals and making communication across the brain faster and more effective. You could think of the locus coeruleus as your brain's master switch, shifting neural dynamics through distinct modes.[87]

When the locus coeruleus is minimally active, as it is during sleep, it plays a crucial role in memory consolidation and recovery, with occasional bursts of activity that help cement the day's learning. As we wake, it shifts into a baseline state marked by low-level activity and a tendency for mind wandering, perfect for creative exploration but less suited to detail-oriented work.

One step above in activity, the brain shifts into a *cruising gear,* producing moderate tonic (background) activity punctuated by well-timed phasic (burst) responses to significant stimuli.

The lower end of this activity range is best suited to routine tasks and task-switching. As it ramps up, this state becomes ideal for focused attention, learning, and complex problem-solving—high engagement without overwhelm.

At peak activity the locus coeruleus floods the brain with noradrenaline, preparing us to face immediate challenges or threats. While essential for intense focus and swift action, lingering too long in this high-alert state can lead to anxiety, fragmented attention, and mental exhaustion.

Cognitive Gears: A New Mental Operating System

The *Cognitive Gears* model helps us recognize these mental states and, more importantly, builds awareness for making intentional shifts into the most effective mode when needed.

I'd like you to imagine that the following three *Cognitive Gears* represent mental states from gentle cruising to high-speed activity.

> **Low Cognitive Gear:** Time in Low Gear is characterized by waking rest and low-level activity. This could include sitting quietly, letting your mind wander, or going for a walk.

> **Middle Cognitive Gear:** Time in Middle Gear is characterized by tasks that require some attention but where we're often switching. During a workday, this could include attending meetings, reading and replying to emails, sending instant messages, and completing small, less complex, lower-priority items on your to-do list.

> **High Cognitive Gear:** Time in High Gear is characterized by being fully engaged, working efficiently and effectively, often on demanding work that requires sustained focus. You might be working on an important new proposal for a client, conducting an analysis, or concentrating on reading and considering the implications of a report, for instance.

Similar to the intensity zone model in endurance sports, you can also imagine a zone above high gear when our brain goes into overdrive, such as in a fight-or-flight response. We'll explore how to manage this mode in chapter 7 because just as cyclists can't maintain zone three indefinitely, our brains aren't designed for relentless high intensity. Our body and brain need strategic shifting between gears to balance effort with recovery to sustain high performance.

Reduce Inefficiency: Cut Down Time in Middle Cognitive Gear

How much time do you spend in each of these *Cognitive Gears* during the average workday? Over the past decade, I've posed this question in hundreds of presentations and workshops. The answer is almost always the same: Most knowledge workers are stuck in *Middle Cognitive Gear*—stuck in unnecessary meetings, feeling like they're on someone else's schedule, with an unspoken pressure to look busy rather than being able to focus on being productive.

So what's the solution? Eliminating all the time spent in *Middle Cognitive Gear* isn't realistic. There will always be small tasks to complete, interruptions to handle, and switching to manage. However, we can significantly reduce our time in this gear. Tackling the overwhelming number of meetings that have crept onto our calendars and improving the efficiency and effectiveness of those that remain is a high-leverage place to begin.

While meetings may be set by employees at all levels, leaders hold the key to reducing the burden of unnecessary meetings, setting the tone for a more focused and productive work culture.

Streamline Your Meeting Calendar

With that in mind, I often encourage leaders to conduct a *calendar purge,* based on the following four steps, to counter the meeting surge many knowledge workers have experienced over the last few years:

Audit Your Meetings: Start by identifying recurring meetings that offer little value. Review your calendar and pinpoint those meetings that consistently feel redundant or unproductive. Ask yourself whether the meeting achieves clear outcomes or if its objectives could be met through alternative methods such as emails or quick check-ins.

Cut the Clutter: Once you've identified low-value meetings, cancel them. These meetings often go unnoticed once they're removed. If you find they were essential, you can always reintroduce them, but many are unlikely to be missed.

Scale Back the Rest: Reduce the frequency of the remaining meetings. If a meeting is weekly, consider shifting it to biweekly or even monthly. Again, there's nothing to stop you from revisiting the schedule and increasing the frequency of some meetings if you find that you need to, but at least it will be a conscious decision rather than being driven by inertia.

Slash Meeting Lengths: I dare you to cut your meeting times by 50 percent and see what happens. Parkinson's Law suggests that tasks expand to fill the time available. Shorter meetings often lead to more focused, efficient discussions. Also, the longer the meeting, the greater the likelihood of multitasking, whereas shorter meetings tend to promote higher engagement.[88]

These steps may seem radical, so I encourage you to approach them as a time-limited team-wide experiment to make the change more palatable. Commit to trying out these four actions and observing the effects for at least eight weeks, then ask everyone on your team to report back and share their experiences.

"This Meeting Should Have Been an Email": Beware the Meeting Maker

You also need to be on the lookout for one of the most disruptive types of knowledge workers: the *meeting maker*.

Meeting makers trigger activity avalanches that cascade through teams, transforming issues that could be addressed in concise written messages into sprawling meetings.[89] Despite representing only 5 percent of the workforce, they can be responsible for generating a staggering 60 percent of all meetings.[90]

Meeting makers also tend to have the worst meeting hygiene—arriving late, allowing discussions to drift, and rarely ending on time.

Short of cutting off their internet access and deleting their calendar accounts, one of the best ways to counter the *meeting maker effect* is by establishing team-wide protocols that require everyone to assess if a meeting is genuinely necessary.

You could consider running another eight-week experiment where all team members are required to answer the following questions before scheduling a meeting:

Have I thought it through? Start by asking yourself if you've fully thought through the situation. If not, schedule time for your own strategic thinking before involving others.

Do I need outside input to make progress? Consider whether you truly need input from others or if existing resources—or even a quick online search—might provide the answers you need.

Do we need a real-time conversation? If you require external input, ask yourself if it necessitates live interaction. If not, an email or another asynchronous method may be more efficient.

What's the most appropriate channel? If a real-time discussion is necessary, decide whether it needs to be face-to-face. If not, an instant message, phone call, or video conference might serve just as well.

What do I need to do to prepare myself and others? When you reach this stage, ensure effective preparation. Set a clear agenda, define your desired outcomes, and distribute any preread materials in advance.

Several organizations I've worked with have codified these steps in a flowchart and distributed them to everyone on the team. Evidence strongly indicates that it's worth the effort. Annual savings from cutting unnecessary meetings are estimated to be around $2.5 million for organizations with one hundred employees and a staggering $100 million for those with five thousand employees.[68]

Four Questions for Meeting Makers

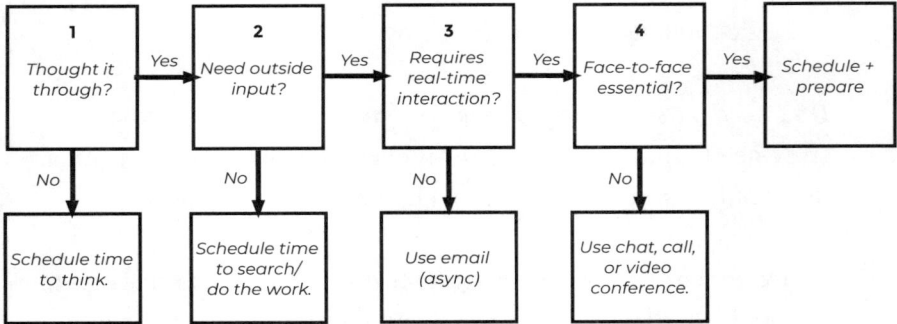

| 1 Thought it through? | →Yes→ | 2 Need outside input? | →Yes→ | 3 Requires real-time interaction? | →Yes→ | 4 Face-to-face essential? | →Yes→ | Schedule + prepare |

No↓ (Schedule time to think.)   No↓ (Schedule time to search/ do the work.)   No↓ (Use email (async))   No↓ (Use chat, call, or video conference.)

Enhance the Quality of the Meetings That Remain

By the end of this process, your calendar should be refined, and only the meetings that truly matter should remain. To ensure these meetings are of high quality, you can apply a simple three-part model centered on purpose, people, and presence.

1. PURPOSE: DEFINE WHAT YOU ARE TRYING TO ACHIEVE

Every meeting should have a clear intent. Consider categorizing meetings into one of the following three types to make the focus of the meeting clear:

- **Decision-Making:** Requires clear ownership and must conclude with concrete choices.
- **Creative Solutions:** Thrive on collaborative energy and generate actionable solutions.
- **Information Sharing:** While sometimes necessary, this final category should be scrutinized most heavily—could the meeting be an email instead?

Success hinges on having a designated *meeting chief of staff* responsible for classifying every meeting into one of the three types, questioning if the meeting is truly required, preparing and distributing materials in advance, and establishing clear ownership of decisions.

2. PEOPLE: DECIDE WHO NEEDS TO BE THERE

Meeting effectiveness depends on role clarity. Every participant should fit into one of the following four categories:

- **Advisers** (who provide strategic input).
- **Recommenders** (who analyze options).
- **Decision-Makers** (who hold the final vote).
- **Execution Partners** (who implement solutions).

Think of these roles as instruments in an orchestra—each plays a distinct part in creating the final symphony. When roles blur, harmony becomes discord. Inefficiency rises, and accountability dissolves.

3. PRESENCE: COMMIT TO FULL ENGAGEMENT

Presence isn't just attending—it's also showing up fully engaged.

- **Silence Digital Distractions:** Turn off notifications and keep phones out of sight and out of reach to stay fully present.
- **Limit Meeting Size:** Smaller meetings encourage active participation—five to seven people is the sweet spot.
- **Engage with Camera Presence:** In virtual meetings maintain eye contact by looking at the lens, not the screen.
- **Facilitate Inclusive Dialogue:** Leaders should actively draw out contributions from every participant.
- **Focus on Quality over Length:** A well-structured twenty-minute meeting often accomplishes more than a two-hour marathon.

Presence is transformative for meeting culture in organizations. A *Harvard Business Review* article provided a great example of what this could look like.[91] A senior leader at a multinational company was renowned for multitasking and never being fully present. In response, he was gently advised to work on this weakness. The leader hired a trainer and developed his mindfulness skills over several months. The result? He ended up being able to reduce the time he spent in meetings by 21 percent(!). Colleagues also rated him as more engaged and pleasant to work with.

Research also indicates that reducing time spent in meetings by 20 percent is associated with an average 26 percent reduction in employee stress and a 35 percent boost in productivity.[92]

Improve Communication Efficiency

Reducing unnecessary meetings is critical in cutting down time in *Middle Cognitive Gear*. However, we also need to take down communication inefficiency. A recent review synthesized twenty-five years of research into *super actions*, which you can use to begin this process.[93]

Break Free from Continuous Communication: When did we decide that email should be treated like instant messenger rather than an asynchronous communication tool?

Instead of constantly checking your inbox, as many knowledge workers do, switch off email notifications and set specific times—such as the start, middle, and end of the day—to process messages. Even if chat notifications remain activated for urgent issues, this *email timeboxing* approach can enhance productivity and lower stress.[94,95]

Focus on What Matters: Approach your inbox with intention. Use a labeling or prioritization system to highlight critical messages and filter out nonessentials. With several AI-powered tools now available, you can streamline and even automate this process for greater efficiency.[73]

Establish Team-Wide Norms: Real gains in communication efficiency emerge when teams adopt these practices. Consider running training sessions to set standardized communication protocols, clarifying the purpose of each communication channel (email, chat, phone, etc.) and offering guidelines on making communication clear, concise, and actionable.

Implementing these steps to minimize time in *Middle Cognitive Gear* can drive impactful results. Meeting purge experiments using similar techniques have saved companies an average of eleven hours per employee each month—equivalent to reclaiming nearly three and a half weeks annually.[96] Streamlined communication strategies can recover a generous portion of the 180 hours knowledge workers lose each year to inefficiencies.[76]

High Cognitive Gear: Enhance Your Decisiveness and Focus

After freeing up a few hours each week from *Middle Cognitive Gear*, consider reallocating some of this time to *High Cognitive Gear*—focused, high-priority work that delivers the greatest impact. Many knowledge workers are surprised by how much they can achieve with just one or two hours of concentrated *High Gear* work a few days each week. The key to maximizing this time lies in identifying when you're naturally primed for complex tasks and efficient, effective work.

Chronoworking: Adapting Work Schedules to Your Circadian Rhythm

Cognitive performance can fluctuate by 20 to 40 percent throughout the day, making certain times better suited to different types of work.[97] The nature of this variation depends on our *chronotype*—our biological tendency toward *morningness* or *eveningness*, as we explored in chapter 1.

Morning types (early birds) typically experience a cognitive *peak* in the early hours of the day, when they feel most alert and focused. This is followed by a midday *valley*, when energy and concentration dip, and then a late-day *rebound*, which brings a lift in energy and attention, though usually not to peak levels.

Early Birds

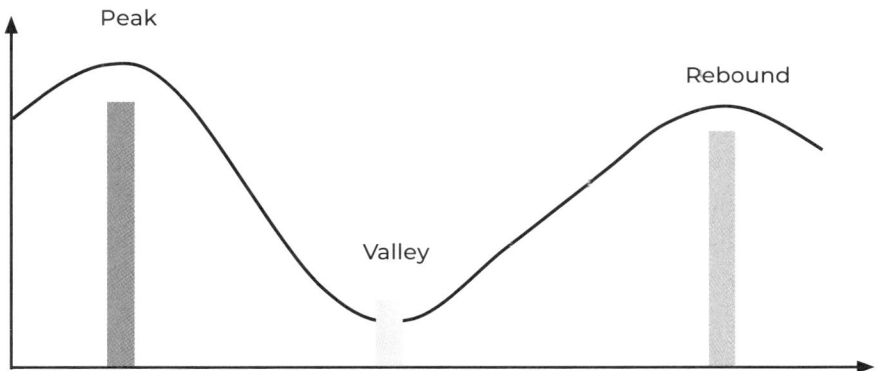

Ana Adan et al. (2012) Circadian Typology

Evening types (night owls), in contrast, experience their *rebound* upon waking as they ease into the day more gradually. They reach a similar midday *valley*, then hit their *peak* in the late afternoon or evening, sometimes extending into the night.

Night Owls

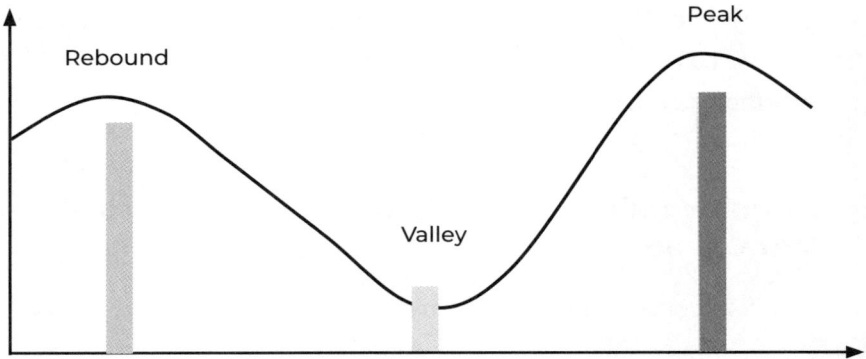

Ana Adan et al. (2012) Circadian Typology

The valley, which often falls after lunch, occurs whether or not we have eaten. It's actually due to a slight discrepancy between the two systems I introduced in chapter 1—the homeostat hourglass timer and the circadian clock. If increasing homeostatic sleep pressure begins to encourage sleepiness before the circadian clock has begun to counteract it, we experience midafternoon drowsiness.[98]

As a result of this variation in cognitive performance and alertness, we have a limited period optimally suited to *High Cognitive Gear* and peak cognitive functioning. Consequently, many knowledge workers benefit from identifying this peak period and allocating it to focus on complex, high-value tasks. The *rebound* period, whether in the morning or later in the day, is better suited to the remaining *Middle Gear* work when switching between smaller, less complex tasks can work well. The *valley* is a great opportunity for *Low Cognitive Gear* recovery, which we'll cover in the next section.

This approach—known as *chronoworking*—structures work to align with natural circadian rhythms, managing energy and boosting focus and productivity. I appreciate that few people have the luxury of aligning their schedules perfectly with their body clocks every day. Nonetheless, I encourage you not to give up on the idea. For example, I've worked with teams who have introduced one meeting-free day each week, allowing employees to work in alignment with their personal rhythms and preferences. Even this small step can make a surprisingly significant positive difference to employees' sense of efficiency, effectiveness, decisiveness, and focus.

Engineer Your Environment for Focus

Now that you've identified your peak period, the next step is to *engineer your environment* to support *High Cognitive Gear* work.

Unfortunately, instead of serving as a sanctuary for sustained attention, our workspaces are often a battleground filled with distractions and interruptions, so it's essential to take the following proactive steps to protect our time in *High Cognitive Gear:*

> **Eliminate Weapons of Mass Distraction:** Start with your biggest culprits—communication tools. During your peak period, commit to switching off notifications and closing email and instant messaging apps. Consider setting an autoresponder to let others know you're available only for genuine emergencies. For an extra layer of focus, place your phone out of sight or, even better, in a different room. Research shows that simply having a smartphone nearby can impair working memory and fluid intelligence by 10 percent.[99] Some people find that blocking software, which limits access to applications that they find particularly distracting, such as social media, can help.

> **Turn Down the Volume:** A noisy work environment can quickly derail productivity. Research shows that a 10-decibel increase in noise—equivalent to turning on a dishwasher or vacuum cleaner—can reduce productivity by 5 percent.[100] Noise is particularly disruptive to detail-oriented tasks—software engineers report more bugs and lower productivity when exposed to background noise.[101] We may not even realize its impact, as noise impairs cognitive performance without increasing our sensation of effort. Invest in quality noise-canceling headphones if a quiet workspace isn't an option.

Turn Up the Lights: There's a strong *dose-response relationship* (where a greater dose leads to a larger effect) between light intensity and alertness—our ability to stay awake, attentive, and responsive.[102] Higher illuminance is also associated with improved cognitive function and attention, so aim to work in a well-lit environment during *High Cognitive Gear* time.[103] Typical office lighting ranges from 90 to 180 lux, but indoor lighting during the day should be at least 250 melanopic equivalent daylight illuminance (melEDI) lux—ideally brighter.[29] As introduced in chapter 1, melEDI lux is a unit of measurement that reflects the effect of light on the human circadian system.

Even sitting near and facing a window, rather than in the center of a room, can make a surprisingly significant positive difference.

Establish Your Priority: Only a small subset—perhaps 2.5 percent of people—are *supertaskers,* able to perform two attention-demanding tasks simultaneously with no performance cost.[104] For the other 97.5 percent, multitasking usually leads to higher stress and diminished results. Most of us, then, are better off focusing on a single task during our *High Cognitive Gear* period. To make the most of this peak time, clarify your priority in advance, ideally the night before. The following tools can help you identify tasks best suited to single tasking.

> **Urgency Importance Matrix:** Use this matrix to prioritize high-importance, low-urgency tasks, making sure they get the focused time they deserve.

> **Action-Priority Matrix:** *High Cognitive Gear* time, which coincides with the peak period in your day, is an ideal opportunity to work on high-impact, high-effort projects, as you will feel naturally more alert and engaged for this more demanding work.

Urgency/Importance Matrix

High

Importance

| Focus | Manage |
| Avoid | Minimize |

Low   **Urgency**   High

Action/Priority Matrix

High

Impact

| Quick Wins | Major Projects |
| "Fill-Ins" | Thankless Tasks |

Low   **Effort**   High

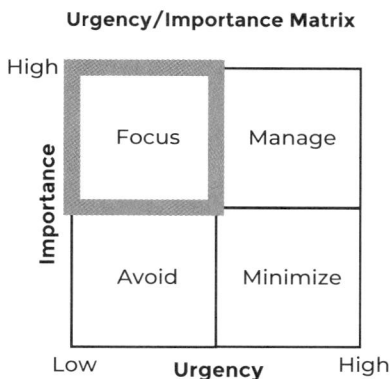

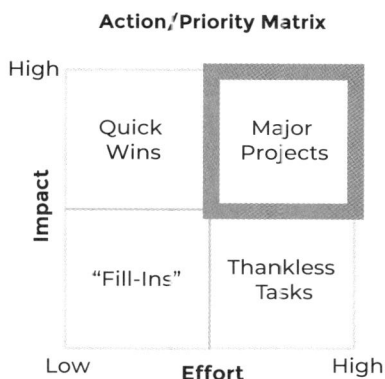

Set a Timer: When people begin to transition out of the constant partial attention that often characterizes knowledge work, focusing for an hour or two can feel overwhelming. In this case, many people find the *Pomodoro Technique*—a time management method developed in the 1980s—helpful. Named after the tomato-shaped kitchen timer (pomodoro is Italian for tomato), this method provides a structured approach to breaking longer periods of *High Gear* work into smaller blocks.

Think of the *Pomodoro Technique* as *interval training for your brain,* with alternating periods of high-intensity work and short, lower-intensity recovery breaks. Start by breaking your *High Cognitive Gear* time into twenty-five-minute focus intervals (each called a Pomodoro), followed by a five-minute break. After three or four cycles, take a longer rest of fifteen to thirty minutes. (We'll explore what to do during the breaks in the next section).

The *Pomodoro Technique* aligns with research on ultradian rhythms, which describe natural cycles of alertness.[105,106] People can generally stay focused for between ten and thirty minutes (depending on the individual) within broader ninety-minute cycles. With all that said, don't unduly restrict yourself to twenty-five- or thirty-minute blocks. If you find yourself in deep focus, feel free to continue without interruption—adapt the structure to suit your natural flow.

Many people find that spending time in *High Cognitive Gear* is not only productive but is much more satisfying, too. There may also be a meaningful commercial impact. Research in firms across five major sectors revealed optimizing knowledge workers' time with dedicated focus periods could be worth $468 billion annually.[76]

Low Cognitive Gear: Reenergize and Recover During Your Workday

We don't think twice about scheduling a meeting in our calendar, but few people plan breaks during their day, even though this simple practice could offer significant benefits.

A practical first step for integrating *Low Cognitive Gear* time into your day is to commit to placing small breaks between meetings whenever possible. The meeting-streamlining techniques introduced earlier can help make this more feasible. While hustle culture may glorify jam-packed calendars, the reality is that back-to-back meetings compromise both well-being and performance.

Here's why and how:

1. OUR BRAIN NEEDS BREAKS

Brain imaging studies provide real-time insights into the cognitive and emotional toll of constant meetings. Recent research compared brain activity in knowledge workers during back-to-back meetings versus when participants took short breaks in between.[107] Continuous meetings were linked to *higher beta brain wave activity*—a neural signature of elevated stress—and *negative frontal alpha asymmetry,* a phenomenon associated with lower engagement. In contrast, breaks between meetings led to *reduced beta activity,* indicating lower stress, and *positive frontal alpha asymmetry,* a marker of higher engagement.

Though the measurement techniques are sophisticated, the message is simple: Our brain needs regular breaks. Far from compromising productivity, these short pauses enhance both well-being and performance.

2. INTEGRATE MICROBREAKS IN YOUR DAY

Evidence is mounting to support *microbreaks*—brief pauses between tasks—as a way to significantly enhance well-being and performance. A meta-analysis of twenty-two studies, encompassing over two thousand participants, found that microbreaks don't reduce productivity, even if they slightly reduce total work time.[108] The time spent on these breaks is compensated by a postbreak improvement in performance. Even pauses of fewer than ten minutes can increase energy levels and reduce fatigue, with microbreaks proving especially effective for reenergizing people when their engagement is low.[109]

Incorporating five- to ten-minute breaks between meetings or tasks is a straightforward yet powerful way to enhance mental resilience and maintain productivity throughout the day.

Once you've committed to integrating a few microbreaks into your day, the next obvious question is: What should you do during the breaks? Consider integrating at least one or two of the following four characteristics:

Relax: Find a way to reduce your cognitive load. This is very intuitive—try to avoid work demands for a while. Adding a laugh can make it even more effective—watching a short comedy clip has been shown to boost cognitive performance by 12 percent afterward.[110]

Socialize: Connect with someone supportive, either in person or digitally. Interaction with a trusted person can lift your mood and make upcoming challenges feel up to 30 percent easier.[111]

Move: A short burst of activity can transform well-being and performance. Brief *exercise snacks* of just two minutes break up long sitting periods, counteracting health risks.[112] For a creativity boost, try a walk outdoors—research shows it can double the likelihood of generating novel, high-quality ideas.[113]

Go Natural: Time in nature is uniquely restorative, as it initiates *effortless attention* in refreshing contrast to the voluntary attention required for work.[114,115] Viewing natural fractal patterns, such as tree branches, stimulates calming alpha brainwaves.[116] Even an indoor garden can cut fatigue, and a mere ninety-second video of a forest scene can trigger measurable relaxation in the brain.[117,118]

Idle Time Is Not a Waste of Time

Regardless of your chronotype, most people experience a dip in energy and alertness around the middle of the day. This *valley* is an excellent opportunity to take a slightly longer break, maybe thirty to sixty minutes. Once upon a time, I believe this was commonly known as a lunch break.

Many driven knowledge workers struggle with the sense that they are losing precious time by taking time off during the day, but our brain does some of its most important creative work when we rest. *Idle time is not a waste of time.*

Creativity is a vital capability in the workplace. It will only grow in importance as routine work is increasingly automated. However, enhancing creativity might require us to do *less work, not more.*

Our brain's most complex, uniquely human parts are engaged during downtime when it is free of inputs and can wander. This activity is described as *random episodic silent thought,* or *REST.*[119] We need time off and *REST* to enable our brains to explore our unconscious reservoirs of thought. When we do, we're more likely to experience the flashes of insight characterizing creativity. So next time you need a breakthrough, your best action might be to take some time out in Low Cognitive Gear.

Earlier in the chapter, I shared research indicating that 22 percent of employees experience burnout symptoms in the average organization.[77] This rate drops to just 2 percent in organizations that prioritize recovery while also seeing a 26 percent boost in performance.[77]

Working smarter works.

Seven Days in Our Cells: The Biological Case for Weekly Rest

In addition to integrating microbreaks and taking a slightly longer break during the valley in your workday, you may also want to consider taking one complete day off each week.

Hybrid working has blurred the boundaries between weekdays and weekends. A survey of more than five thousand workers who work at least four days per week, with at least one of those days at home, found that 54 percent worked at least six hours on Saturday or Sunday.[120]

This is not necessarily a problem—10 percent of the respondents reported not working on any given weekday, so this weekend work likely reflected people taking advantage of hybrid-working flexibility. But it's also possible that, for some people, this trend reflects an unhelpful breakdown of work-life boundaries. If you choose to work on the weekend, no problem. If you feel compelled, it may be more of an issue.

There may still be a case for everyone taking one day off in seven, though.

In addition to our daily *circadian rhythm,* our bodies may have a weekly rhythm. Approximately seven-day cycles known as *circaseptan rhythms* are observed across a remarkable range of living things—from single-celled organisms to humans. You can imagine them like a weekly metronome, which influences everything from our blood pressure and heart rate to our immune system and stress hormones.[121,122]

The evidence for these weekly rhythms is still emerging and less robust than that for well-established biological rhythms, such as the 24-hour circadian cycle. Nonetheless, it remains intriguing. Many of these seven-day patterns persisted when researchers placed people in caves or special facilities cut off from all external time cues—no clocks, calendars, or social schedules. This suggests they're not simply a product of our modern weekly calendar—even though this plays a role—but something that may have a basis in our biology.[121,122]

It's also interesting to note that historical attempts to alter the seven-day week have consistently failed. When revolutionary France tried to implement a ten-day week and when the Russian revolution attempted a five-day week, their experiments collapsed because of widespread physical and psychological strain among workers.

These historical accounts and our growing scientific understanding of *circaseptan rhythms* suggest something profound: Our bodies may be biologically programmed to operate optimally on a seven-day cycle.

The science of *circaseptan rhythms* is far from definitive. Still, it offers a fascinating insight that might explain why seven-day weeks and the practice of taking one day of rest have emerged across various cultures and have proven so enduring. If you're not in the habit of taking one day off in seven, I encourage you to try it.

Find and Follow Your Rhythm

While *always-on work* pushes us toward constant activity, our biology appears to be insisting on a different rhythm—one that combines effort with recovery as a necessity rather than a luxury. In this context it's clear that *hustle culture* runs counter to how our body and brain are wired. At the same time, *quiet quitting* swings too far the other way—rediscovering more natural rhythms of work and rest can help us meet work demands without burning out.

Both *hustle culture* and *quiet quitting* also rest on the false belief that well-being and performance are at odds. In reality, rhythms of deliberate, efficient, focused work paired with effective rest form the foundation for sustained high performance, individually and organizationally.

Knowledge work is a *cognitive endurance activity.*

CHAPTER 2 REVIEW

In this chapter we explored how knowledge work has become increasingly demanding on our minds, with calendars overloaded by meetings and constant connectivity disrupting focus. I introduced a new framework—*Cognitive Gears*—to help structure workdays more effectively, drawing parallels between athletes' endurance training and knowledge work performance.

KEY INSIGHTS

THE CURRENT STATE OF KNOWLEDGE WORK

- Weekly meetings have increased by 153 percent.
- Knowledge workers spend 10 percent of their time toggling between applications.
- Interruptions strike every eleven minutes, with refocusing taking up to twenty-three minutes.
- A total of 54 percent of workers feel compelled to signal their presence even when not working.

UNDERSTANDING COGNITIVE GEARS

- **Low Gear:** Characterized by waking rest and low-level activity.
- **Middle Gear:** Task-switching, meetings, emails, and routine work.
- **High Gear:** Fully engaged, focused work requiring sustained attention.
- Most knowledge workers spend too much time stuck in *Middle Gear*.

MEETING EFFICIENCY FRAMEWORK

- **Purpose:** Define clear meeting types (decision-making, creative solutions, information sharing).
- **People:** Clarify roles (advisers, recommenders, decision-makers, execution partners).
- **Presence:** Ensure full engagement and participation.

CHRONOWORKING PRINCIPLES

- Cognitive performance can fluctuate 20 to 40 percent throughout the day.

- Peak periods are best suited for complex, high-value tasks.
- Valley periods are ideal for *Low Cognitive Gear* recovery.
- Rebound periods work well for *Middle Gear* tasks.

PRACTICAL ACTIONS

1. STREAMLINE YOUR MEETINGS

- Audit recurring meetings for value.
- Cut unnecessary meetings.
- Scale back meeting frequency.
- Slash meeting lengths by 50 percent.

2. ENGINEER YOUR ENVIRONMENT FOR FOCUS

- Turn off notifications during *High Gear* work.
- Use noise-canceling headphones if needed.
- Ensure adequate lighting (minimum 250 melEDI lux, but ideally more).
- Remove distracting devices.

3. INTEGRATE RECOVERY PERIODS

- Schedule short breaks between meetings.
- Take a proper lunch break during your valley.
- Include some form of movement in breaks.
- Consider taking one complete day off each week.

Remember This

Knowledge work is a cognitive endurance activity. Like physical training, sustainable performance requires the right mix of intensity, recovery, and attention to natural rhythms.

Looking Ahead

In our next chapter, we'll explore how to improve our ability to unwind and disconnect from work.

CHAPTER 3

REGENERATIVE DOWNTIME: IMPROVE YOUR ABILITY TO UNWIND

It feels like we are *always on,* but the more we need to switch off from work, the harder it becomes.

Four experiences are vital for effective *recovery* from work—which describes the process of restoring our physical and mental energy reserves.[123]

Control: Deciding *your* schedule and what you want to do.

Detachment: Gaining a sense of mental distance from work.

Mastery: Learning new things and broadening your horizons.

Relaxation: Taking it easy and making time for leisure.

However, in an era of constant connectivity, the lines between the personal and professional have all but disappeared. What was once time for winding down and recharging at the end of the day is now regularly interrupted by work demands.

Consider the data: Rather than feeling in *control,* 55 percent of employees say they experience pressure to answer calls or check emails outside of working hours. *After-hours work*—defined as working past 5:00 p.m.—has risen by 28 percent.[67] Only 45 percent of employees report feeling able to disconnect from work.[124]

Rather than feeling a sense of *detachment,* people are finding it increasingly difficult to disconnect. A total of 72 percent of employees report worrying about work during their downtime, and one-third say that simply thinking about work disrupts their work-life balance more than the actual work itself.[125, 126, 127]

Longer workdays leave little room to expand our perspectives, cultivate *mastery,* or enjoy the restorative benefits of learning and engaging in other fulfilling activities. All our eggs are increasingly in the basket of work.

In search of respite and *relaxation,* many knowledge workers turn to distractions, hoping to carve out a sliver of me time. Yet in doing so, they often fall into the trap of *revenge bedtime procrastination*—extending their evenings and sacrificing sleep to reclaim the leisure time they lost during the day.[128] Others turn to alcohol in the hope that it will help them unwind, without realizing that this perceived psychological benefit comes at the cost of huge disruptions to the restorative quality of sleep.[129]

This cycle reveals a paradox—the times when recovery from work is most needed are precisely when it is hardest to achieve.[130]

Beyond Extremes: Finding Balance in an Always-On World

Knowledge workers are responding to this erosion of boundaries between work and life in polarized ways.

On one side, we find *hustle culture* advocates who believe that boundaryless work is the pathway to success and that replying to an email at 3:00 a.m. is something to be proud of.

On the other side, we find the *quiet quitters*—those who have made a deliberate decision to do the minimum to meet their job description—who wouldn't even consider checking their inbox outside their contracted hours.

Both responses are understandable, yet there is a *third* way—a new approach that sidesteps the extremes of relentless hustle or rigid disengagement. This third way acknowledges the unsustainable demands of hustle culture and the risks of burnout. It also recognizes that the unshakable enforcement of work-life boundaries can have unintended consequences for both employers and employees.

This *third way* also appreciates that condemning after-hours work as universally bad is too simplistic. While some people need to disconnect completely to recharge, others are comfortable working during their free time and may even find it easier to relax if they've ticked off a few tasks in the evening.

There is no one-size-fits-all solution.

As discussed in earlier chapters, adopting a shoshin mindset—a beginner's mind—can help us experiment with new postwork rituals and discover what works for us.

The first step in this process is recognizing how our preferences and predispositions can influence our experience of *control*—deciding *your* schedule and what you want to do.

Control: Are You an Integrator, a Segmentor, or a Vinaigrette?

People vary widely in how they navigate the boundaries between work and personal life. Some prefer a clear divide, taking an *oil-and-water* approach to keeping work and home separate. Others favor a *smoothie method*, blending it all together. But many of us fall somewhere in between—a state best compared to a *vinaigrette*, where constant effort is required to keep the mix together.

Researchers describe these preferences along a continuum, from *high segmentation* (those who prefer strict separation) to *high integration* (those who fluidly blend work and home life).[131] Where we fall on this continuum shapes how we structure our daily routines and perceive the relationship between work and home.

The Work-Life Segmentation Spectrum

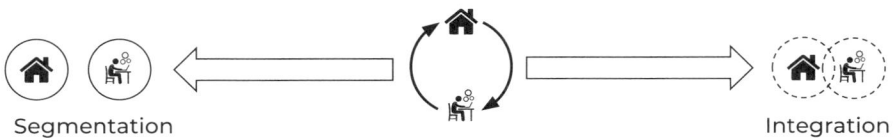

Segmentation ← → Integration

Integrators tend to see space and time as flexible, assigning roles and activities without rigid boundaries. They're less likely to distinguish between personal and professional identities—parent, friend, or employee—and find it natural to check work emails over dinner or handle personal matters during the workday. For *integrators,* this fluid approach brings a sense of control and reassurance. Ironically, doing some work after hours can help them gain a sense of mental distance from work and unwind. For *integrators,* this experience of after-hours work could be described as problem-solving pondering, which involves reflecting on work and exploring potential solutions to challenges in a way that is positive and rewarding.[132,133]

Integration can also accommodate a greater diversity of personal needs and preferences. For example, some people may take a break in the afternoon, whether for exercise, the school run, or something else, before putting in a *second shift* later in the day.

Integrators also transition smoothly between roles, experiencing less stress when moving from professional to personal tasks. However, *role confusion* is the potential downside of this blurred boundary. Prioritizing can become challenging, and conflicts may arise, especially if a partner with a strong preference for segmentation expects undivided attention at home, for example.

Segmentors prefer clear boundaries between work and personal life, ensuring that each role remains distinct. For them, work tasks—such as responding to emails—are meant for the office, not the dinner table. This approach helps *segmentors* avoid the feeling that they should be on call after hours, but it can come with downsides. For instance, *segmentors* are more susceptible to technostress, finding that after-hours emails or video calls intrude on their personal space.[134]

By focusing on one role at a time, *segmentors* minimize conflict between personal and professional demands, enhancing their ability to stay present in each setting. However, this rigid separation can make transitions feel more disruptive; shifting from work mode to home life requires effort and adjustment. It also limits flexibility, as strict boundaries make it harder to respond to unexpected demands that fall outside designated work hours.

Whether we're consciously aware of it, *integrators, segmentors,* and those of us who oscillate between the two in the *vinaigrette shaker of life* all tend to employ boundary management strategies—techniques that help control the relationship between our personal and professional lives. These strategies fall into the following four main categories[135]:

1. **Communicative** (setting expectations with others).
2. **Technological** (using devices or apps to manage access).
3. **Temporal** (organizing time to reinforce boundaries).
4. **Physical** (arranging spaces to create distinct environments).

Imagine a busy manager who prefers to keep personal matters out of their work life (*high work segmentation*) but is comfortable letting work creep into family time (*low personal segmentation*). They may prefer not to talk about their personal life with colleagues (a *communicative* tactic) and use two phones—one for work, which they always carry, and one for personal life, which they switch off while working—to keep work and home separate (a *technological* tactic). However, lower family segmentation preference means they are happy to catch up on emails in the evening at home (a *temporal* tactic).

In contrast, some people focus more on keeping work from intruding on family time (*high family segmentation*) but don't mind personal and professional blending at work (*low work segmentation*). Imagine a project manager who works from home, is happy for family photos to be seen in the background of his video calls, and often completes a few household chores in breaks during the day but who is very strict about switching off his work phone at 6:00 p.m. to enjoy uninterrupted family dinners (a *temporal* tactic). To manage this, he sets clear expectations with his boss and colleagues about his no-work-after-hours rule (a *communicative* tactic) and switches off notifications to ensure this is adhered to (a *technological* tactic).

Problems Arise When Strategies Are Blocked and Boundaries Erode

Tensions can surface when people are unaware of others' work-life segmentation preferences, preventing them from using the boundary management strategies they rely on to gain a sense of control in an *always-on* work culture.

Leaders, in particular, can create pressure on their teams to work against work-life segmentation preferences without realizing it. For example, managers and senior employees are often inclined to work in the evenings and on weekends.[136] They may be entirely comfortable with this approach, especially if they are *integrators* who naturally blend work with personal life.

However, working and sending after-hours messages can implicitly signal that round-the-clock availability is expected of everyone, regardless of their preferences or personal circumstances, even if that's not the intent.

Research into how managers' and leaders' communication patterns influence their teams underscores this effect: Every hour a manager works after hours leads to an additional twenty minutes of after-hours work for all their direct reports.[136]

Issues can also emerge when employees are too rigid in their boundary management. For example, the same employees who will not work a minute after 5:00 p.m. should not necessarily expect their employer to be flexible during the workday if they need time off for personal reasons.

Psychological Detachment: Everyone Needs to Switch Off, but It's Hard

Regardless of our preference for *integration*, *segmentation*, or the *boundary management strategies* we employ, *psychological detachment*—the experience of switching off and gaining a sense of mental distance from work—is essential for recovering from work and for health and well-being more broadly.[137,138] When people struggle to let go of work-related thoughts, their psychological stress response remains engaged. This phenomenon often manifests as affective rumination, which describes persistent worries, tension, and irritation about work.[133] The inability to mentally disconnect from work also carries physiological costs. Elevated levels of stress hormones, such as cortisol, hinder recovery and gradually erode resilience, potentially disturbing sleep and even increasing the risk of health issues such as cardiovascular disease.[139, 140, 141, 142, 143, 144, 145] It's no surprise that constant work connectivity can double work-related stress and burnout rates.[71]

Psychological detachment acts as a mental brake, enabling knowledge workers to switch off and recover both psychologically and physically.[137,146,147] However, technology makes it increasingly difficult to disconnect.

Technology Makes It Difficult to Detach

It was much easier to switch off from work when computers were the size of a conference room. A total of 99 percent of work was done at an office desk between 8:00 a.m. and 5:00 p.m. Employees might bring home a few documents to read, but with rare exceptions, there was no expectation of communicating outside normal working hours. Out-of-office really meant out of touch, and the boundaries between work and home life were clear.

This norm shifted in the late 1980s when mobile technology became cheaper and more ubiquitous. First came pagers—pocket devices that beeped or vibrated to let you know you had a message, usually with a phone number to call back. Then came home computers with internet connectivity. Eventually, laptops and smartphones meant that we could stay connected and keep working anywhere, anytime, making it almost impossible to leave work behind.

Beware the Zeigarnik Effect and Ironic Rebounds

Many of us end the day feeling like our minds are browsers with too many tabs open. This experience can be amplified by the *Zeigarnik effect,* which describes how the thoughts of all the tasks we haven't completed occupy our minds significantly more than those we've finished.[148]

Unfortunately, trying to stop thinking about these unfinished tasks will likely have the opposite effect to the one we're hoping for.

Before we continue, I have an important request:

> *As you read this, try not to picture a bright pink elephant. Whatever you do, don't imagine the pink elephant standing in a field, wearing sunglasses, waving its trunk at you. Just focus on the words here and avoid picturing that pink elephant.*

What are you thinking about now?

This corny exercise makes an important point. Trying not to think about a pink elephant made it much more likely that an image of this animal came to mind. This is an example of the *ironic rebound* effect—trying to suppress thoughts makes them more persistent.

But not everyone seems to struggle equally with psychological detachment. Have you noticed how some people easily leave work behind while others have difficulty, no matter how much (or little) they have left to do?

Just as people differ in their preference for work-life *segmentation* or *integration*, some are naturally more inclined to ruminate—getting caught in cycles of dwelling on thoughts.[137]

This tendency to ruminate is shaped by a mix of biological, psychological, and environmental factors. Yet as we'll explore later in this chapter, whether you're prone to high or low rumination, there are strategies to help improve your ability to detach and unwind from work.

Mastery: Limited Time Can Make Us One-Dimensional

When work dominates our lives, we risk putting all our psychological eggs in one basket—a phenomenon researchers call *reduced self-complexity*.[149] Having multiple, distinct facets to our identity—such as being a musician, a parent, a volunteer, or a professional—provides a natural buffer against stress and setbacks. But in an *always-on* work culture, this resilience is eroded, and we risk becoming one-dimensional.

Engaging in activities that foster *mastery* outside work—those that challenge us, teach us new skills, and build competence—can act as an antidote, enriching our sense of self and bolstering recovery. Yet for many knowledge workers, increasingly limited downtime makes it difficult to prioritize these nonwork pursuits. *Hustle culture* even suggests that time spent outside work is a distraction, overlooking the profound value of nonwork activities.

Instead of learning a new language, taking up rock climbing, or perfecting a creative skill, too many knowledge workers remain tethered to their professional identities, sacrificing both psychological recovery and personal growth.

Relaxation: There's a Battle for Your Downtime

Never mind pursuing new hobbies and developing our sense of self—many knowledge workers would settle for some time to chill out.

Relaxation—taking it easy and making time for leisure—is the most intuitive aspect of recovering from work, yet this experience remains out of reach for many. Long days and after-hours work erode opportunities to switch off, leaving little time to unwind. In response, people are looking for quick fixes.

For many, the evening routine has been reduced to collapsing on the sofa and switching on a favorite show, letting the plot sweep them into another reality. Watching something to help you relax is harmless enough most of the time, but not always.

Imagine the scene: You've finally settled onto the sofa after a long day. You want to unwind but still get an early night, so you tell yourself, "Just one episode." But as the episode wraps up, the main character teeters on the edge of a cliff-hanger. What happens next?

Autoplay has already queued up the next episode. It's tempting, especially when you can skip the intro and dive right into the action. You convince yourself you'll only watch a few more minutes just to close the loop so you don't go to bed worrying about the ending. But soon, you decide to watch the whole of the next episode, reasoning that after such a demanding day, you've earned it—a classic case of *revenge bedtime procrastination*.

Let's be honest. It's never *"just a few minutes."* One episode turns into another, and then maybe a few minutes of the next, until good intentions evaporate, and another hour or two of sleep slips away. It's no accident. Senior executives in the streaming industry have admitted that sleep is their biggest competitor—these platforms are designed to keep us hooked.[150]

The Happy Hour Trap: When Unwinding Becomes a Habit

While some people unwind by binge-watching series, others try to shortcut relaxation with alcohol.

Despite a decline in popularity, particularly among younger employees, many knowledge workers still turn to alcohol as a way to decompress and psychologically detach from work.[151,152,153] The ritual of coming home—or stepping away from the home office—and reaching for a beer or pouring a glass of wine remains deeply ingrained. In fact, knowledge workers consume about 20 percent more alcohol than other occupational groups.[154]

In the short term, this approach may appear effective. Alcohol stimulates the release of a neurotransmitter cocktail of dopamine, gamma-aminobutyric acid, serotonin, and endorphins, leading to feelings of elation and relaxation.[155,156]

Alcohol also has a *biphasic effect*. Shortly after drinking, alcohol levels in the bloodstream begin to rise, creating a stimulating effect that boosts mood and fosters a sense of positivity.[157,158] Assuming we don't continue drinking, our blood alcohol level declines as the body metabolizes the alcohol. This gradual descent in alcohol concentration brings a sedative effect, which we often interpret as relaxation and the sense that we stop overthinking.[155,156]

Unfortunately, overrelying on alcohol to unwind can trap some people in a harmful cycle. Even modest consumption—about 0.25 grams of alcohol per kilogram of body weight (equivalent to roughly a glass and a half of wine or two beers for a 165-pound [75 kg] person)—can reduce physiological recovery during sleep by nearly 10 percent.[129] Poor sleep, in turn, elevates stress the next day, making it harder to relax without another drink.[159] This disrupted cycle of poor recovery and rising stress can quickly become self-reinforcing, creating a vicious cycle.

I conducted a study as part of my academic research to compare the physiological and psychological effects of drinking alcohol after work. The data made it clear that any perceived psychological upside was overwhelmed by the physiological downside in terms of impaired recovery.[79]

The implication is clear: We need to find healthier approaches to unwinding that truly restore us. This process can begin by identifying our preferences for work-life segmentation.

Improve Your Sense of Control: Identify Your Work-Life Segmentation Preference

Being able to live and work in perfect alignment with our preference for either *segmentation* or *integration* is unlikely—and arguably, such rigidity might not even be healthy. However, identifying our preferences and employing supportive *boundary management strategies* can lay the groundwork for greater control and more effective recovery from work.

You can measure your *work-life segmentation preference* using the following scale, originally developed by Organizational Psychologist Glen Kreiner.[131]

On a scale from 1 to 7 (1 = *strongly disagree*, 4 = *neutral*, 7 = *strongly agree*), indicate the extent to which you agree with the following four statements:

I don't like to have to think about work while I'm at home.	1	2	3	4	5	6	7
I prefer to keep work life at work.	1	2	3	4	5	6	7
I don't like work issues creeping into my home life.	1	2	3	4	5	6	7
I like to be able to leave work behind when I go home.	1	2	3	4	5	6	7
Average:							

Calculate Your Score

Average Your Ratings: Sum the ratings for all four statements, then divide the total by 4 to calculate the average.

Interpretation: Higher scores (on a scale from 1 to 7) reflect a greater preference for segmentation and vice versa.

For example, if someone answered 6, 5, 5, 6, this would result in an average of 5.5, indicating a relatively high preference for segmentation. Many people find it helpful to complete this survey with friends, family, and colleagues to better understand each other's preferences.

Designing Boundary Management Strategies to Support Your Work-Life Balance

Once you've identified where you fall on the segmentation-integration spectrum, the next step is to consider how *boundary management strategies* can support your preference and provide a sense of *control* in your experience of recovery from work. For example:

Communicative Strategies: Setting Expectations

Clear communication can be one of the most powerful tools for reinforcing your boundary preferences. If you lean toward *segmentation*, share your preference with colleagues or clients. Set an automatic reply stating your working hours and usual response times if possible. This simple step can reset expectations, prevent misunderstandings, and begin to reduce after-hours work. For *integrators*, open communication can also be helpful—for example, letting your team know that you're available for quick questions via chat in your free time but that you may not respond to emails immediately. Communicative boundaries also extend to family and friends, who may need reminders about work times if you work from home. You could also set expectations concerning exceptions—such as using phone calls for emergencies during what would typically be a "do not disturb" time, for example.

Technological Strategies: Using Devices and Apps to Control Access

Technology can help or hinder boundary management. *Segmentors* can take advantage of features such as Focus Mode on smartphones and laptops or app blockers that limit work-related notifications during scheduled times. *Integrators,* on the other hand, might set up focused notification systems that allow only high-priority messages to come through after hours, ensuring they stay informed without overwhelming personal time. The delay send feature in email clients is another useful tool for both preferences; it allows you to work on messages when convenient but ensures they're delivered during regular hours to accommodate colleagues with differing preferences.

Temporal Strategies: Structuring Your Time

Temporal strategies involve organizing your time to align with your boundary preference. *Segmentors* might set designated work hours and avoid scheduling work tasks during evenings or weekends. This structure helps them switch off mentally and signal to others when they are available. For example, blocking off your calendar after 6:00 p.m. and silencing notifications helps establish a consistent boundary. *Integrators,* in contrast, might prefer time-blocking techniques that allow for shorter work bursts interspersed with personal activities.

For instance, if you're an *integrator*, you could dedicate specific times for personal errands or family calls within the workday, striking a balance without disrupting productivity.

Physical Strategies: Creating Distinct Spaces

Physical boundaries offer another effective way to separate work and personal life. *Segmentors* could create dedicated spaces for work, such as setting up an office area they leave once work hours are over. This helps reinforce the mental shift between roles. Even small changes, such as closing the door to your workspace or moving to a different room, can enhance this effect. On the other hand, integrators may find it helpful to use transitional items to adjust between roles—such as a favorite coffee mug for work hours and a different one for personal time. Simple cues, such as changing into more casual clothes after finishing work tasks, can serve as signals that help reinforce a smoother transition.

How Leaders Can Support Healthy Boundaries and Resilience

Leaders, in particular, must recognize how their actions can conflict with team members' preferences and undermine their boundary management strategies. Many leaders' fondness for after-hours communication often stems from habit or outdated assumptions that long hours are a proxy for productivity rather than genuine necessity.

Providing employees with a sense of control over how they approach work demands can be a powerful buffer against high job pressures and significantly support recovery. In a study analyzing twenty years of mental health and medical data from over three thousand individuals, researchers found that when job demands were high but employees had low control, the risks of depression and all-cause mortality (the likelihood of dying from any cause within a given period) rose sharply.[160] However, when employees had a stronger sense of control, their physical health improved—even when job demands remained high.

It's also worth noting that a survey of thirty-two thousand people across twenty-eight countries found that 80 percent of employees expect company executive to model healthy behavior, particularly in setting and respecting work-life boundaries.[161] This is an important reminder of leaders' critical role in fostering a culture that respects and supports sustainable working habits, enabling people to experience a sense of control and switch off when needed.

Clear communication about control and flexibility expectations is essential, and flexibility should work both ways. Neither employers nor employees can predict every demand life will throw at them, and rigid boundaries may not always be realistic. Ideally, a foundation of trust and respect allows for mutual flexibility: Employees may occasionally need to adapt to work requirements outside their usual preferences for *segmentation* or *integration*, while employers should respect their team's ability to structure time and energy in ways that align with those preferences most of the time. This mutual understanding fosters a balanced and adaptable workplace where all parties feel supported and empowered.

Improve Your Ability to Psychologically Detach

Leaders can play a key role in helping employees manage boundaries and switch off from work, but we can also take personal steps to improve our ability to *psychologically detach*. Observing the habits of *low ruminators*, who naturally find it easier not to dwell on work-related thoughts, is a good place to begin.

Low ruminators are typically proactive about *boundary management*.[137] For instance, they might leave their phone in another room when spending time with friends or family. *Low ruminators* also actively engage in tactics to avoid rumination rather than hoping unwinding will occur spontaneously. For example, *low ruminators* might schedule a conversation with a friend or plan a social activity after work, which can help shift their thinking away from professional responsibilities.

In contrast, *high ruminators* can be their own worst enemies.[137] They often keep their smartphones close by, making it harder to truly switch off. When troubled by persistent negative thoughts, they often withdraw from social contact, even though time with others might be exactly what they need to *get out of their heads*.

While alone time can help us recharge, social interaction is critical to human well-being and performance. Chapter 8 of this book features a deep dive into the importance of *relatedness*—our innate need for social connection.

Landing the Day: Easing into Detachment from Work

Even if we apply these *boundary management strategies,* improving our ability to psychologically detach from work can still feel like a paradox—the harder we try, the more elusive it becomes, thanks to the ironic rebound effect—remember the pink elephant?

Many knowledge workers need to rethink how they think about work.

Psychological detachment is less like flicking a switch and more like landing a plane. Attempting a rapid descent can lead to a bumpy rebound, where work thoughts resurface just as we try to relax. A smoother transition involves gradually reducing mental speed and altitude, easing ourselves away from work mode.

For some, socializing after work offers this soft landing, providing an effortless shift in focus. Others benefit from a structured process that guides them from rumination to *problem-solving pondering mode* before mentally switching off. You can think of this transition as a prelanding routine—a few proactive steps that help shift the mind from work to rest, paving the way for a more successful, stress-free landing into relaxation.

Problem-solving pondering still involves thinking about work. However, rather than dwelling on uncomfortable emotions, problem-solving pondering is more constructive. And unlike rumination, which drains energy and hinders recovery, problem-solving pondering can be restorative.[132,162]

Next time you find yourself stuck at thirty-five thousand feet in a rumination-holding pattern, struggling to land your metaphorical mental plane, try switching your thinking into *problem-solving pondering mode*. Practically, this can involve shifting our mind from thoughts that increase tension and negative emotions to more solution-oriented actions. For example, if you notice you are ruminating on a work-related issue, try to think of one useful action you can take at that moment, even if it doesn't fix the situation immediately. This could involve writing a brief list of the actions you can take to resolve the issue or simply blocking some time in your calendar to work on the problem the following day.

Counter the Zeigarnik Effect by Making a Plan

As I mentioned earlier in this chapter regarding the *Zeigarnik effect,* sometimes the thought of unfinished tasks troubles us the most. Creating a plan to tackle the issue can help you stop thinking about it, even though it remains unfinished. Research suggests that the more specific the plan, the easier it is to detach from the thoughts.[163]

This approach can also help us shift *emotion to action*. Some of the most difficult thoughts to let go of often relate to emotions. Our *why-related* thoughts are often the most sticky and emotional. For example, you might find yourself repeatedly thinking, *Why am I always the one who has to take responsibility?* in relation to a work colleague and experiencing unpleasant emotions related to this. If you're feeling stressed about an emotive topic and struggling to switch off, take a moment to pay attention to your thoughts and notice if there are any *why* thoughts hanging around.

Shifting *why* thoughts to *how* actions can make them less sticky and easier to let go. Again, we can do this by thinking, and perhaps even writing down, one useful action we can take. For instance, if you kept thinking, *Why am I always the one who has to take responsibility?* you could write a note reminding yourself to schedule a time to speak with your team about how actions and responsibilities are being allocated.

Implementing proactive boundary management strategies, postwork unwinding rituals, and techniques to counter rumination could measurably improve your ability to psychologically detach, with a wide range of additional benefits. Higher levels of psychological detachment are associated with improved mood, better sleep quality, and reduced fatigue, especially under high job demands.[164] Contrary to what the *hustlers* may tell you, switching off from work actually boosts productivity: Employees who limit after-hours work are, on average, 20 percent more productive.[71]

Even though they may be comfortable with integration, leaders still benefit from detaching from work. Recent research highlights that continually thinking about work can diminish leaders' effectiveness.[165] In contrast, leaders who were better able to psychologically detach from work felt more energetic and were more likely to inspire and motivate their teams.[165]

Recharge Your Mind with Mastery Experiences

Engaging in activities that foster *psychological detachment* can also spark a positive cycle, freeing up mental energy for other enriching pursuits. This could include activities that provide experiences of *mastery*—the sense that we are learning and growing, ideally while doing something unrelated to work.[166] Investing time and energy outside work also allows us to diversify our identity so we aren't putting *all our eggs in one basket*. This broader sense of self can enhance resilience, making us less vulnerable to work-related stress.[149]

Sport and exercise are particularly effective for promoting *mastery*, as they can provide a sense of clear progress, in stark contrast to knowledge work, where this experience can be rare. Exercise can also significantly reduce stress and increase psychological detachment from work.[167, 168, 169, 170] Exercise has even been explored as a substitute for alcohol. Researchers hypothesized that a brief workout could replicate some of alcohol's effects by triggering a similar release of neurotransmitters. The results were compelling: A short exercise session significantly reduced alcohol cravings, lifted mood, and lowered anxiety, highlighting exercise as a powerful tool for mental recovery and well-being.[171]

There are many ways to experience *mastery* beyond exercise, though. Spending time pursuing almost any self-directed activity that promotes creativity and freedom can significantly improve measures of well-being.[172] For instance, creating *visual art* such as painting, drawing, or photography can positively influence resilience and reduce negative stress. This effect was highlighted when researchers evaluated the effects of a ten-week visual art intervention on brain activity, focusing on the default mode network—a network of brain regions that become particularly active when our minds are at rest.[173] This mode of brain activity was more strongly associated with stress resistance after participants actively produced art rather than passively evaluating it. This suggests that making art could improve our stress resistance and ability to recover from work.

If you haven't already, I encourage you to consider how you might incorporate *mastery experiences* into your free time—opportunities to learn something new, take on fresh challenges, and expand your horizons.

Develop a Personalized Relaxation Tool Kit

Sometimes, going to the gym, pursuing a hobby, or pulling out our paints feels like too much effort. I get it. In this case, I encourage you to find a healthy way to unwind, ideally without alcohol. I still enjoy a glass of wine or a beer. However, being aware of the negative effects on recovery, I drink less and favor quality over quantity, both in what I drink and who I drink with. For those of us who enjoy the ritual of a postwork beer, nonalcoholic options are also getting better all the time. You can also consider experimenting with the following alcohol-free ideas to help you relax after work:

Pace Your Viewing

Watching a favorite show can be a great form of escapism and relaxation. However, instead of binge-watching, experiment with limiting yourself to one episode per evening. Turning off the *autoplay* feature—which usually can be found in the settings on the browser version of streaming apps—has been a game changer for many people trying to slow their series consumption. This small bit of friction, where we need to select the next episode consciously, can create just enough pause to help us do the right thing, turn off the screen, and head to bed, avoiding revenge bedtime procrastination and encouraging us to savor a series over time.

Dim Your Space to Signal Relaxation

A few subtle changes to your environment can encourage natural relaxation. Dim lights to 10 lux or lower (lux is a unit of measurement for light intensity) in the three hours leading up to sleep.[174] Switching to warmer, amber, or red-toned lighting also promotes relaxation, setting a gentle mood that cues sleepiness. Various smart bulbs and home lighting systems are available to facilitate this.

Unwind with Slow-Tempo Music

Many people have experienced the relaxing benefits of music. Listening to slower tempo tracks—around fifty-six beats per minute—can improve mood and reduce stress. Just twenty minutes of listening has been shown to raise *oxytocin* (a hormone linked to feelings of connection and trust) and increase *heart rate variability*, a marker of *rest-and-digest* activity in the nervous system, while lowering heart rate.[175] Several music platforms let you search for songs by tempo, providing the opportunity to curate a personalized playlist of slow-tempo tracks to add to your relaxation tool kit.

Take a Breath: The Science of Using Paced Breathing for Relaxation

When you're feeling stressed or struggling to relax, has anyone ever told you to just "take a breath"? It may sound like clichéd advice, but this suggestion has a strong neurophysiological basis. Consciously pacing our breathing can shift brain activity and adjust physiological responses to promote relaxation, improve mood, decrease blood pressure, and reduce cortisol levels.[176,177] Many of these effects relate to the structure and function of the vagus nerve—a long bundle of nerve fibers that starts in the medulla oblongata, a part of the brain that controls many of the body's most important functions—before passing through the heart, lungs, and ending in the large intestine.

The vagus nerve makes up 75 percent of the parasympathetic *rest-and-digest* branch of our nervous system.[178] When we breathe slowly, the rhythmic expansion and contraction of our lung tissue increases the activity of the vagus nerve.[179,180] This increase in activity shifts the nervous system toward a parasympathetic *rest-and-digest* state and away from a sympathetic *fight-or-flight* state.[181] Slow, controlled breathing can also change electrical activity patterns in the brain via the vagus nerve, increasing power in *alpha band* brain wave frequencies and decreasing *theta power*, which is associated with reduced tension and anxiety.[182,183]

Providing you don't have any underlying health conditions associated with breathing or heart function, many people find the following breathing exercise helpful:

1. Find somewhere comfortable where you can lie down or recline. This allows your diaphragm, the muscle that controls breathing, to move easily.
2. Start by taking a comfortable breath through your nose. There is no need for a deep or large breath.
3. Next, exhale slowly until your lungs feel comfortably empty before inhaling normally. Over the next few breaths, gently bring your attention to your breathing.
4. Try to breathe through your nose as much as possible.
5. As you breathe in, gently shift your breath from your chest to the abdomen. Feel your abdominal muscles expand as you inhale

and contract as you exhale. If it's helpful, imagine that there is a balloon in your abdomen. As you inhale, gently inflate the balloon. As you breathe out, gently let the air out of the balloon.

6. Continue this pattern for two to three minutes, breathing at a pace of around six breaths per minute—inhaling for a count of five and exhaling for a count of five.

7. Notice the sensations of your breath passing in and out of your nose.

This technique may not feel natural initially, and you may need to concentrate, but the effort should be cognitive, not physical. Don't try to pull air in or push air out. Allow the air to pass in and out of your lungs.

Breathing practices may not always feel relaxing. If you feel tense or worried during the exercise, notice and accept how you feel. There is no right or wrong sensation. If you feel anxious, let go of your intention to relax and gently shift your focus to the breathing process.

Breathing exercises may not work for everyone, but some evidence indicates that regular slow breathing practice over three months can lead to durable shifts toward parasympathetic rest and digest dominance.[181] Over time, this simple slow breathing technique might become a helpful tool for shifting your nervous system and relaxing your mind.

Reflecting on Recovery: Using Measurement to Guide Improvement

As a final step, you can use the Recovery Experience Questionnaire, developed by Sabine Sonnentag and Charlotte Fritz, to identify whether there is an aspect of recovery that you may benefit from emphasizing.[123]

On a scale from 1 to 5 (1 = *I do not agree at all* to 5 = *I fully agree*), indicate the extent to which the following sentences accurately describe your experience and activities during your free time.

CONTROL					
I feel like I can decide for myself what to do.	1	2	3	4	5
I decide my own schedule.	1	2	3	4	5
I determine for myself how I will spend my time.	1	2	3	4	5
I take care of things the way that I want them done.	1	2	3	4	5

Control Average: (*Calculate the average of your responses to the control statements.*)

DETACHMENT					
I forget about work.	1	2	3	4	5
I don't think about work at all.	1	2	3	4	5
I distance myself from my work.	1	2	3	4	5
I get a break from the demands of work.	1	2	3	4	5

Detachment Average: (*Calculate the average of your responses to the detachment statements.*)

MASTERY					
I learn new things.	1	2	3	4	5
I seek out intellectual challenges.	1	2	3	4	5
I do things that challenge me.	1	2	3	4	5
I do something to broaden my horizons.	1	2	3	4	5

Mastery Average: (*Calculate the average of your responses to the mastery statements.*)

RELAXATION					
I kick back and relax.	1	2	3	4	5
I do relaxing things.	1	2	3	4	5
I use the time to relax.	1	2	3	4	5
I take time for leisure.	1	2	3	4	5

Relaxation Average: (*Calculate the average of your responses to the relaxation statements.*)

CALCULATE YOUR SCORE

Calculate Averages: For each category (*control, detachment, mastery, and relaxation*), add up your scores and divide by the number of items in that category to find the average.

Interpreting Results: Higher averages indicate a stronger presence of that characteristic in your free time activities. For example:

A high *control* average suggests that you feel autonomy in managing your time.

A high *detachment* average indicates effective separation from work during free time.

A high *mastery* average shows that you actively seek growth and challenge.

A high *relaxation* score suggests a strong tendency toward unwinding and relaxation.

While higher scores indicate a stronger recovery experience in that area, lower scores may highlight aspects of recovery worth prioritizing.

In Summary

Work can feel relentless, but as this chapter has shown, practical, evidence-based strategies can help you reclaim downtime and boost recovery. I encourage you to consider which approaches might enhance your unwinding routine. By consciously integrating experiences of *control*, *detachment*, *mastery*, and *relaxation* into your postwork rituals, you can survive and even thrive amid the demands of *always-on* work.

CHAPTER 3 REVIEW

In this chapter we explored why disconnecting from work is becoming increasingly difficult despite our growing need for recovery. We examined the four vital experiences needed for effective recovery—*control, detachment, mastery,* and *relaxation*—and discovered practical strategies to improve our ability to unwind in an always-on world.

KEY INSIGHTS

UNDERSTANDING WORK RECOVERY

- **Control:** Deciding your schedule and activities.
- **Detachment:** Gaining mental distance from work.
- **Mastery:** Learning and broadening horizons.
- **Relaxation:** Making time for leisure.

WORK-LIFE INTEGRATION STYLES

- **Integrators:** Blend work and personal life fluidly.
- **Segmentors:** Prefer strict boundaries between work and home.
- **Vinaigrettes:** Oscillate between integration and segmentation.
- Each style requires different boundary management strategies.

BOUNDARY MANAGEMENT STRATEGIES

- **Communicative:** Setting expectations with others.
- **Technological:** Using devices/apps to manage access.
- **Temporal:** Organizing time to reinforce boundaries.
- **Physical:** Arranging spaces to create distinct environments.

EVENING RELAXATION TOOLS

- Pace viewing your favorite shows instead of binge-watching.
- Dim lights to 10 lux or lower before sleep.
- Use slow-tempo music to aid relaxation (around fifty-six beats per minute).
- Practice controlled breathing exercises.

PRACTICAL ACTIONS

1. ASSESS YOUR WORK-LIFE STYLE

- Complete the work-life segmentation preference scale.
- Calculate your average score.
- Identify boundary management strategies that match your style.

2. MEASURE YOUR RECOVERY EXPERIENCE

- Use the Recovery Experience Questionnaire.
- Calculate scores for control, detachment, mastery, and relaxation.
- Identify which aspects need more attention.

3. DEVELOP A PERSONALIZED RELAXATION TOOL KIT

- Choose screen time management strategies.
- Create an environment conducive to unwinding.
- Practice the breathing exercise provided.
- Consider alternatives to alcohol for relaxation.

Remember This

Recovery from work isn't a luxury—it's essential for sustainable performance. The key is finding strategies that align with your personal preferences for managing work-life boundaries.

Looking Ahead

In our next chapter, we'll explore how to improve our sleep quality without becoming obsessed with sleep optimization.

CHAPTER 4

REGENERATIVE SLEEP: HOW TO CARE ABOUT SLEEP WITHOUT OBSESSING

Despite our growing knowledge and increasing investment in sleep, restful nights elude many of us.

The *sleep economy*—which spans smart mattresses, wearables, supplements, and coaching—is booming.[184] Over one-third of people have tried a sleep-tracking device.[185] But paradoxically, this increasing focus on sleep doesn't seem to be helping. Around 30 percent of adults report sleep problems.[186] So what can we do about it?

The conundrum of sleep is that we can't simply *will* ourselves into a better night's rest. In fact, the more effort we invest, the further peaceful slumber seems to drift out of reach. Still, that hasn't stopped people from trying.

The Hyperoptimizers: Making Sleep a Competition

In addition to prescribing rigid morning routines, a growing faction of *hyperoptimizers* seems intent on turning sleep into a competitive sport, complete with supplement regimens, elaborate protocols, and *biologically plausible* justifications for everything. The introduction of *sleep scores* on wearable devices—metrics that claim to quantify sleep quality—and the rollout of *sleep challenges* have only fueled this trend. Wearables have long told us who's running farther or cycling faster; now they reveal that our friends and colleagues are supposedly better at sleeping, too.

The Sleep Deniers: They Think Short Sleep Is Still Something to Boast About

At the opposite end of the spectrum are the *hustle culture* advocates who still believe that not sleeping enough is something to be proud of. Jokes about being "too busy to sleep" and war stories about all-nighter work sessions abound. These sleep deniers transform what should be warnings about unsustainable work practices into symbols of dedication and excellence, convinced they are immune to the effects of sleep deprivation.[187,188]

The Quiet Quitters: Improving Sleep Feels Too Tiring

Between the *hyperoptimizers* and the *hustlers*, we once more find the *quiet quitters* ensnared in the *triangular relapse pattern* that I described in chapter 1. They begin with a newfound commitment to sleep, adopting a carefully crafted routine with enthusiasm. But when life inevitably disrupts their plans, maintaining this overly ambitious regimen becomes exhausting. Frustrated, they slip back into old habits, abandoning hope that their sleep will ever improve—until the next game-changing sleep protocol appears on their social media feed, prompting them to start the cycle anew.

We Need to Avoid These Extremes

Ideally, we'd approach healthy sleep without slipping into the traps of obsessing like the *hyperoptimizers,* ignoring it like the *hustlers,* or giving up like the *quiet quitters.* This balanced path begins by adopting a shoshin beginner's mindset. As you read this chapter, I invite you to explore the concepts you'll encounter with openness and curiosity, setting aside rigid preconceptions or fixed ideas about sleep. We'll start by examining why sleep can be such a challenge, tackle common questions, debunk a few popular myths, and then end with practical strategies to support healthy sleep without it becoming yet another source of stress.

The Problem Began with Electric Lights

Why do so many of us struggle with something that should be so natural?

In chapter 1 I introduced our brain's master clock—*the suprachiasmatic nucleus*—a structure that keeps us in sync with the earth's twenty-four-hour rhythm through inputs from light-sensitive cells in our eyes.

For the vast majority of human history, the sun served as the primary light cue for the suprachiasmatic nucleus, anchoring a stable rhythm as day transitioned predictably into night. The advent of electric lighting changed everything. Unlike its predecessors—fire, candles, and lanterns—electric light more closely mimicked sunlight and extended illumination well beyond sunset, disrupting the natural balance of light and dark.

This revolutionary lighting paved the way for our 24/7, *always-on* world. Untethered from the sun's rhythm, we could eat, work, and play at any hour. The seamless harmony between our internal clock and the earth's light-dark cycle faded. Bedtimes and waking, once instinctive, now require conscious control—a skill we continue to struggle with.

Approximately 70 percent of people experience irregular sleep and wake patterns because of social jetlag—a mismatch between our internal body clocks, work obligations, and social schedules.[189] Globally, an estimated 45 percent of the population may be sleep deprived.[190,191,192,193] Without consistent cues from the natural environment, the concept of healthy sleep has become increasingly elusive, leaving many unsure about when they should go to bed, wake up, and how much sleep they truly need.

How Much Sleep Do We Need?

You don't need to be a sleep scientist to recognize that some people need more sleep than others. If people can sleep for as long as they wish, most reach a stable sleep duration of around eight hours (eight and a half for younger adults and seven and a half for older adults).[95]

Plotting self-reported sleep duration on a graph reveals a bell-shaped *normal distribution*. You can see seven to eight hours in the middle of the curve, representing the average for most people. The majority fall within one *standard deviation*—a way to measure how spread out a set of numbers is—on either side of this average.[194]

The distribution's tails are at either end of the curve—people who report six hours or fewer at one end and those who sleep nine hours or more at the other—but these extremes are rare. The weight of evidence and expert consensus strongly supports the view that adult humans need between seven and nine hours of sleep to maintain health and quality of life.[195,196]

Normal Distribution in Sleep Duration

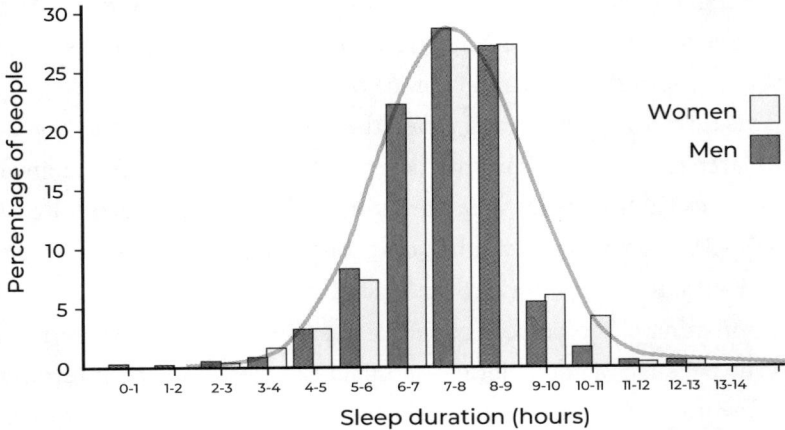

Figure adapted based on Groeger et al. (2004)

Whenever I present these findings, I'm often asked about people who seem to get away with sleeping very little. Individuals with a mutation on a gene—DEC2—involved in regulating the circadian clock and the sleep-wake cycle seem more resistant to the effects of short sleep.[197,198,199] This mutation is exceptionally rare, with estimations that it occurs in 0.02 percent of the population.[200,201] To provide a practical sense of what that means, in a five-thousand-seat concert hall, one person might be carrying this genetic mutation.

The DEC2 mutation represents a genetic exception, not a strategy that others can replicate. Most people who sleep little and believe it doesn't affect them are likely unaware of the extent to which their performance is impaired. A sleepy brain is similar to a drunk brain, making us very poor judges of how we are functioning.

The Hidden Toll: We Don't Notice Sleep Deprivation's Impact

Several studies reveal that our perception of sleepiness tends not to correlate with changes in our performance. Hans Van Dongen, a sleep scientist, and a group of researchers carefully controlled the sleep duration of healthy participants for fourteen consecutive days and nights. The participants were randomized to sleep for either four, six, or eight hours per night. A fourth unfortunate group was completely deprived of sleep for three nights.

The researchers observed the participants and measured their cognitive performance during their waking hours. Sleeping six hours per night for two weeks was associated with impairments in cognitive performance equivalent to going two nights without sleep.[202] However, when the researchers analyzed the participants' self-reported perception of how alert or sleepy they felt, some curious findings emerged.

The participants whose sleep was restricted to four hours or fewer felt progressively sleepier and foggy throughout the study. In contrast, the participants who slept for six hours per night initially felt slightly sleepier, but this perception soon plateaued. Meanwhile, their performance continued to deteriorate. The participants' perceptions became detached from reality, meaning they were largely unaware of how sleeping six hours per night negatively affected them. Impaired performance became their new normal.

More recent research by Melissa St. Hilaire and colleagues investigated a variable pattern of sleep restriction alternating between severe restriction (three hours) and recovery (ten hours).[203] This variability more closely mimics real-world scenarios where people oscillate between sleep loss and longer recovery sleep.

The findings confirmed that subjective sleepiness ratings did not match objective performance impairment, reinforcing the dangerous disconnect between how sleepy people feel versus their actual impairment. The researchers also discovered that despite apparent recovery after ten-hour sleep opportunities, the benefits were temporary—performance deteriorated more rapidly when subjects were rechallenged with sleep restriction.

The results of both studies highlight that sleep-deprived people consistently underestimate their impairment levels. Further, the discovery that recovery sleep provides less protection than previously assumed challenges the popular strategy of compensating for sleep loss with occasional long nights of sleep.

Can We Adapt to Shorter Sleep?

The lack of awareness of how short sleep impairs us may explain why several prominent influencers continue to promote *core sleep*—an outdated and debunked idea that we can adapt to sleeping four and a half to five and a half hours, perhaps topped up with a few naps. Social media algorithms often amplify these claims as they promote engagement and debate, but the popularity of the posts is misleading—most represent a complete misunderstanding and misinterpretation of scientific evidence.

While some older studies suggested that sleeping four and a half to five and a half hours could support satisfactory performance, this research related to performance in repetitive tasks was based on very structured sleep schedules, often in extreme contexts such as single-handed oceanic sailing races, over limited periods.[204,205] Adopting a core sleep approach disrupts circadian rhythms and results in missing a huge amount of rapid eye movement (REM) sleep, which is essential for learning and memory. It is not a suitable method for squeezing more hours out of the average day.

Sleeping fewer than seven hours each night significantly impairs complex cognitive capabilities such as problem-solving, decision-making, emotional intelligence, and socio-emotional processing, which are critical for performance at work and in our personal lives.[206,207,208] Advocates of short sleep also rarely address its negative impact on long-term health.

Adequate Sleep Is Foundational for Physical and Mental Health

Regularly sleeping fewer than seven hours per night is associated with a range of health risks, including an increased likelihood of developing cardiovascular and metabolic diseases such as coronary heart disease, diabetes, and some cancers.[196]

Not sleeping enough also impairs our immune system. For example, sleeping fewer than seven hours can increase the risk of developing a common cold by 300 percent.[209] In addition, not sleeping enough can lead to unhealthy behaviors. In one intriguing study, researchers set up a supermarket and monitored purchases made by participants on a fixed budget, comparing their behavior when they were sleep deprived with when they had slept adequately.[210] Sleep-deprived participants purchased nearly 10 percent more calories than when they were well rested, as their appetite regulation was impaired.

Inadequate sleep is also associated with worse mental health.[196] Many of us will have noticed that stress can lead to sleep problems.[211,212,213] If you've ever lain in bed staring at the ceiling while *ruminating* (struggling to stop thinking), you know what I mean. Chapter 3 includes several ideas that could help put the brakes on rumination. Chapter 7 will tackle the topic of stress management specifically.

While the relationship between stress and sleep is often discussed, it's less well known that it is *bidirectional*.[159] While stress can interfere with sleep, not sleeping enough can elevate stress. This effect is likely related to changes in *amygdala* activity—a brain structure responsible for processing our emotions.[214] Shortening sleep can heighten activity in the amygdala and amplify our stress responses. Many high-quality studies have highlighted the importance of sleep for emotional well-being. In fact, sleep is so critical for our mental health that some researchers have characterized sleep as *overnight therapy*.[207] Sleep's effect on our ability to process emotions and on our reactions also has significant implications for how we interact with each other in a business context.

Want to Build a High-Performing Team? Start with Sleep.

While sleep is becoming a huge topic of interest in the mainstream media, business management education remains largely silent on the subject.[215] Nonetheless, the evidence is increasingly clear that sleep is the foundation for many critical leadership capabilities. For example, when leaders' sleep is restricted to five hours, their problem-solving ability could be impaired, their IQ could decrease by fifteen points, and team members are likely to perceive them as less inspirational and charismatic, as their communication appears less authentic.[202,216,217]

Hustlers and sleep deniers might also want to rethink their celebration of all-nighters. Working for eighteen hours without sleep—equivalent to starting at 7:00 a.m. and continuing to 1:00 a.m.—is associated with declines in cognitive performance equivalent to a blood alcohol concentration of 0.05 percent.[218] That's enough to be arrested for drunk driving in most countries.

Disrupted Sleep Impairs Creativity

In contrast, adequate sleep supports vital capabilities such as creativity. During sleep, we cycle through distinct phases and stages: rapid eye movement (REM) and non-rapid eye movement (NREM) sleep. NREM is further divided into N1, N2, N3, and N4 stages, each leading to progressively deeper sleep. Both REM and non-REM sleep stages play critical roles in creativity.[219]

Sleep Stages

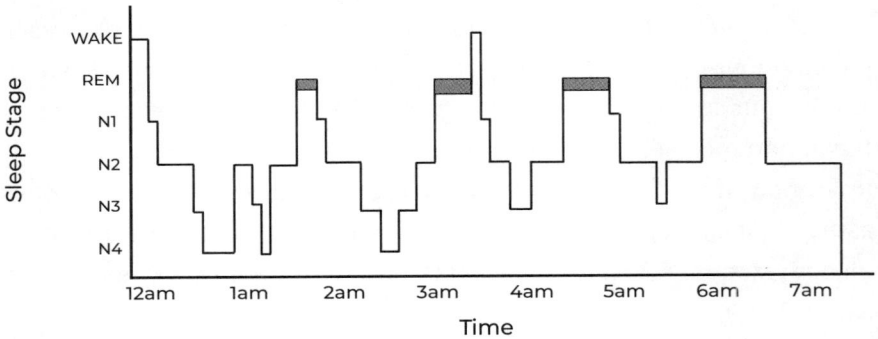

Figure adapted based on Dumay et al. (2005)

Non-REM Sleep distills the essence of related memories, helping us uncover overarching patterns and rules. Think of it as the stage where your brain sifts through the day's experiences to find the golden nuggets of wisdom. On the other hand, REM sleep—characterized by high excitation and connectivity in the brain—is when the creative magic happens. This sleep stage allows your brain to form new, unexpected connections within existing knowledge.

The interplay between REM and non-REM sleep throughout the night enhances our ability to form complex knowledge frameworks, boosting creativity. However, shortened, irregular sleep disrupts this process.

Devaluing Sleep Negatively Affects Teams

Leaders' attitudes to sleep can also affect their employees' sleep and performance. Teams whose leaders encouraged poor sleep habits, such as praising people for all-nighters and demanding instant email responses at all hours, slept for almost half an hour less than people in teams whose leaders demonstrated that they valued sleep.[220] Leaders' *sleep devaluing* attitudes negatively affect employees' sleep quality, increasing the likelihood of team members behaving less ethically.[220] This may relate to the observation that poor sleep impairs the function of the prefrontal cortex—the brain region most responsible for the exercise of self-control.[221]

These impairments have a tangible economic impact. Even without accounting for the impact of clinical sleep disorders, it's been estimated that Canada, the United States, the United Kingdom, Germany, and Japan lose a combined $680 billion every year because of insufficient sleep.[222]

The next obvious questions are, If sleep is so vital, how do we determine how much we truly need, and what steps can we take to support and improve it?

Are You Getting Enough Sleep?

If you're curious about how much sleep you need, answering the following questions is a good starting point.

One: Can you wake up in the morning, close to when you need to get up, without an alarm?

Two: Can you get through an average day without feeling sleepy and relying on stimulants such as caffeine or stress—which many people use as a stimulant without realizing it—to stay awake?

Three: Do you struggle to fall asleep and nap during the day?

If your answer to all the questions is yes, you're probably getting enough sleep. If you answer no to one of them, you will probably benefit from sleeping more.

Does Sleep Need Change as We Age?

As people age, particularly after sixty, their sleep patterns noticeably change. These shifts can include taking longer to fall asleep and waking up more frequently, resulting in shorter, lower-quality sleep.[223]

As with teenagers, aging shifts the interaction between the two systems that regulate sleep and wakefulness: the sleep timer and the circadian pacemaker. However, while this shift pushes teenagers toward later sleep and wake times, in older adults, it narrows the "sleep window" for quality sleep and causes them to wake earlier within their circadian cycle.[3]

The function of our homeostatic hourglass timer also worsens, possibly because the number of *adenosine* receptors in our brain reduces over time, making older adults less sensitive to accumulating sleep pressure.[223] Factors such as weight gain and obstructive sleep apnea may also contribute to disrupted sleep.

While it is not entirely clear whether these changes reflect a reduced need for sleep as we age, it is apparent that our ability to sleep alters. And even if older adults need slightly less sleep, the evidence strongly suggests that adequate sleep, which generally falls between seven and nine hours, remains critically important across our lifespan. Consequently, while both older and younger adults would benefit from paying attention to actions that support healthy sleep, these actions may become even more important as our biological capacity to sleep changes.

Engineer Your Environment to Support Healthy Sleep

The sleep market and social media are obsessed with optimizing sleep through elaborate protocols, high-tech devices, and specialized supplements, but the most effective steps are often the simplest. These are sometimes described as *sleep hygiene practices*.

1. USE LIGHT (AND DARKNESS)

The first step in improving sleep begins long before we head to bed— we need to reintroduce more natural light-dark rhythms into our days.

Morning: Try to wake up at a consistent time each day.

Daytime: Prioritize bright light exposure during the day—this is essential for maintaining a healthy circadian rhythm. Aim to be in environments with at least 250 melEDI lux on the vertical plane at eye level (e.g., sitting and facing a window, even on a cloudy day). Natural daylight is the best option, even if the sky is overcast.[29]

Evening: We should aim to reduce our light exposure in the hours leading up to bedtime. In the three hours before you go to bed, limit light exposure to 10 melEDI lux or less. You can often achieve this by dimming lights and using lights with warmer (orange and red) hues.

Night: During sleep, your bedroom should be as dark as possible, not exceeding 1 lux. As a rule of thumb, if you can see the outline of your hand in front of your face in your bedroom when you are trying to sleep, your room is probably too bright. Darkening a room to 1 lux or less often requires blackout curtains and minimizing electronic light sources, such as the LEDs on devices or switches.

If you can't block out light in the room, consider using a sleep mask to block light from your eyes. This could improve sleep quality[224] and even enhance aspects of cognitive function, such as learning and alertness, the following day.[225] If you need to get up at night, the lights should be kept dim and warm toned (orange and red).

2. BE MINDFUL OF ELECTRONIC SCREENS AND LIGHT AFTER DUSK

It is widely reported that using smartphones and screens before bed negatively impacts sleep. However, varying interpretations of the evidence on the relationship between technology use and sleep have left many people confused.

Articles and social media posts often cite research showing that evening screen use suppresses melatonin levels. While this is accurate, many studies measuring these biological effects did not evaluate their direct impact on sleep.[226,227]

When sleep is measured, the effect on sleep duration may not be as significant as commonly assumed. For example, a review of eleven international studies found that screen use increased the time it took to fall asleep by a maximum of 9.9 minutes.[229] However, to put this into perspective, some commonly prescribed insomnia medications reduce sleep onset latency by only nine minutes.[228]

The relationship between screen use and sleep is also bidirectional. Highly engaging content may tempt people to delay sleep to continue watching, while others turn to smartphones or tablets to relax or pass the time when they struggle to fall asleep.[229]

These findings have led some to question whether the effects of melatonin suppression, light exposure, and technology use before bed are truly significant. In my view, while the delay in sleep onset associated with screen use may be less dramatic than anticipated, its impact can still be meaningful for some individuals. Moreover, evidence strongly suggests that light exposure should be restricted to 10 lux or lower during the three hours before bedtime and avoided entirely at night, as it acts as an unnatural biological signal during these periods.[29]

Finally, removing technology from the bedroom may help reduce potential sleep disruptions for certain individuals. This simple adjustment could support healthier sleep patterns and reinforce better habits over time.[229]

3. MAKE YOUR ROOM AS QUIET AS POSSIBLE

In addition to making our bedrooms as dark as possible, we would also benefit from making them quiet. Nighttime noise can lead to lighter sleep, more awakenings, and changes in sleep stages, leading to poorer sleep quality overall.[230] Noise during sleep can also cause stress responses in the body, including increases in heart rate, elevated blood pressure, and raised stress hormones, even if we don't wake up fully.

As a guideline, the World Health Organization suggests that nighttime noise levels outside bedrooms should be below 40 decibels. This is the sound level you would expect in a quiet library. If you can't soundproof your room sufficiently, consider using earplugs.

4. KEEP YOUR BEDROOM COOL

Our body temperature naturally drops as we approach sleep. A cooler room helps facilitate this process. Ideally, we would control bedroom temperature to between 60°F and 67°F (15.6°C–19.4°C). Infants and elderly people may need slightly warmer temperatures, around 65°F to 70°F (18.3°C–21.1°C). Some people prefer temperatures at the lower or higher end of these ranges, but temperatures above 71°F (21.6°C) or below 54°F (12.2°C) are likely to cause sleep disturbances for most people. It's also worth considering how bedding could contribute to overheating. Thick blankets or warm pajamas might require a cooler room temperature.

If you're used to a warmer room and think you may benefit from cooler temperatures, gradually lower the temperature over a few nights to allow your body to adjust. Ensuring the room is well ventilated to reduce the accumulation of carbon dioxide and keeping humidity between 30 and 50 percent can also contribute to comfortable, quality sleep.

I encourage you to experiment with these ideas and see if they improve your sleep. You can get a sense of whether they are working simply by asking yourself the three questions I posed earlier: Is it easier to wake up without an alarm at roughly the time you need to? Can you get through the day without feeling sleepy and relying on stimulants?

Consistent Sleep Is Critical

It's probably clear by now that most of us would benefit from aiming to sleep for at least seven hours per night. However, the regularity of our sleep and wake times also plays a key role in our health and performance.

Our body and brain work best when we go to sleep and wake up on a consistent schedule. Regular sleep schedules have many benefits, including improved alertness, cardiovascular and metabolic health, lower inflammation, better mental health, improved cognitive performance, and longer and higher-quality sleep.[26]

In contrast, irregular sleep schedules are associated with worse health outcomes, including higher cholesterol and elevated blood pressure.[231] The associations remain even after adjusting for average daily sleep duration, suggesting sleep irregularity is an *independent risk factor* for poor health.

Around 70 percent of people experience *social jetlag*—a difference in the timing of the midpoint of sleep between work and free days—of at least one hour.[189] Many people experience more disruption.[189] Take the following sleep schedule, which imagines a person continually adjusting their schedule around work demands and their social life.

NIGHT OF	BED TIME	WAKE TIME (NEXT DAY)	SLEEP DURATION (HOURS)	SLEEP MIDPOINT	NOTES
SUNDAY	23:15	07:15	8	03:15	Working from home so later start.
MONDAY	23:00	07:00	8	03:00	Sleep consistent with work schedule.
TUESDAY	23:30	06:00	6.5	02:45	Working from office so earlier start.
WEDNESDAY	00:00	06:00	6	03:00	Watched extra episode so later to bed.
THURSDAY	00:30	06:00	5.5	03:15	Late night due to socializing.
FRIDAY	00:30	8:30	8	04:30	Lie in at the weekend.
SATURDAY	01:00	8:12	7.2	04:36	Late night due to socializing.

You can determine social jetlag by calculating the following:

1. The average midpoint of sleep for *weekdays*.
2. The average midpoint of sleep for *weekends*.
3. The difference between these two averages.

In the example above, the average midpoint of sleep on weekdays is 02:45. The average midpoint of sleep on weekends is 04:33. Therefore, their *social jetlag* is 1 hour and 48 minutes.

How to Counter Social Jetlag

Ideally, we would try to keep social jetlag to twenty minutes or fewer. However, even reducing it to under one hour represents a significant improvement for most people and still offers considerable health benefits.

If you're far from this target, view reducing *social jetlag* as a gradual process—trying to make big jumps toward consistency often fails. Instead, aim to reduce social jetlag by maybe twenty to thirty minutes first, then continue making small adjustments as they become sustainable. Any reduction in social jetlag is better than no reduction.

Consider creating incentives that motivate you to adjust your sleep schedule in favor of consistency. For example, planning a Saturday morning brunch can encourage you to go to bed earlier on Friday night, making it easier to wake up refreshed the next day.

As suggested in the previous chapter, turning off the *autoplay* feature on streaming services reduces the temptation to binge-watch, helping you stick to a sleep schedule. Setting a nightly alarm as a cue to start winding down can also be effective, gently signaling it's time to prepare for rest. Adults need bedtimes, too.

I appreciate that many people struggle to sleep enough at consistent times during the workweek. While it's clear that we would benefit from sleeping seven hours per night on a regular schedule, a recent expert consensus offers hope. Sleeping longer on the weekend can help—one to two hours of extra sleep on days off can reduce some of the health risks associated with shorter sleep during the workweek.[26]

How to Counter Travel Jetlag

There's nothing like traveling to throw a spanner in the works of a carefully crafted sleep schedule.

I've been privileged to deliver keynotes and consult for companies all over the world. One particularly intense period saw me speak at nine events on four continents in four weeks. Thankfully, my jetlag was minimal, but this wasn't by chance.

Travel-related jetlag occurs when our internal body clock is out of sync with the local time at our destination due to rapid travel across time zones. However, following some simple science-backed principles can accelerate our adjustment and minimize this disruption.

Managing light exposure and controlling caffeine intake and naps can help your body adapt to a new time zone much more quickly and reduce symptoms such as fatigue and disorientation. The challenge is figuring out when to apply these strategies—timing is critical. Also, some intuitive actions—such as trying to adapt to the new time zone as soon as you get on the plane or getting bright light as soon as you land—can make jetlag worse.

I rarely recommend apps or products, but in this case I'll make an exception—the results have been so overwhelmingly positive for myself and many people I work with. For any trip involving a time zone shift of more than three hours, I always use an app called TimeShifter®.

The app massively simplifies the jetlag mitigation process by allowing you to input your flight details and receive a personalized plan tailored to your sleep patterns and travel schedule. It also provides real-time notifications to guide you on what to do and when—such as when to seek light or avoid caffeine—making it easy to follow a structured plan and minimize jetlag. You can find TimeShifter® in most app stores.

What Can Parents of Young Children Do About Disrupted Sleep?

For parents, taking a trip and experiencing a bit of jetlag might sound like a luxury. While I appreciate this doesn't apply to everyone, the stress and exhaustion from children interrupting sleep can feel overwhelming for many people. If you can relate, offering yourself grace during this challenging time is essential.

Many parents experience periods of sleeplessness with their children. While it may seem never ending in the moment, most children eventually settle into more stable sleep patterns as they grow.

Most importantly, remember that the body's resilience is profound. While chronic sleep deprivation should be addressed, short-term disruptions are not likely to cause lasting harm. If you're struggling, I encourage you to seek support from an appropriately qualified sleep consultant or a health-care provider who can provide reassurance and help establish strategies that promote better sleep for both you and your child.

While sleep is crucial for health, we humans are adaptable. Compassionate, consistent support during this time will help both you and your child regain restful nights.

How the Menopause Transition Can Affect Sleep

Perimenopause and menopause are natural transitions, but they can significantly affect sleep quality for many women. Up to 69 percent of women report experiencing sleep disturbances during the menopause transition.[232] The hormonal changes accompanying menopause—including declines in estrogen and progesterone—can disrupt normal sleep-wake cycles. Additionally, many women struggle with temperature regulation during this time, finding it difficult to cool down at night, which is essential for restful sleep.

There are several strategies to help manage sleep problems during the menopause transition, each targeting different aspects of this life stage. However, I strongly suggest that you seek advice from an appropriately qualified professional before implementing any changes.

Hormone replacement therapy (HRT)—after consulting a health-care provider to evaluate its suitability, HRT can be effective for some women experiencing hot flashes and night sweats, also known as *vasomotor symptoms.*

Cognitive behavioral therapy for insomnia (CBT-I), a form of talk therapy that addresses the thoughts and behaviors contributing to sleep problems, is often recommended as the first line of treatment for women diagnosed with insomnia during menopause.

Digital CBT-I, which provides therapy through online platforms, may offer a more convenient option for those who cannot access in-person treatment.

Sleep hygiene practices, including the tips that I shared earlier, such as going to bed and waking up at the same time every day and creating a cool, comfortable environment for sleep, can help.

Regular exercise can also improve sleep quality, especially if sessions are completed outdoors, as natural light exposure can help regulate the sleep-wake cycle.

For managing hot flashes, lightweight, breathable sleepwear and moisture wicking bedding can reduce discomfort.

Melatonin, a hormone that helps regulate sleep, can improve sleep quality for some women. Still, its effects vary from person to person, and it should only be taken after consulting a health-care provider.

Avoid triggers such as alcohol and smoking that can worsen menopausal symptoms.

While sleep issues are common during menopause, effective treatments are available. I'm aware that this is an incredibly brief section on a very important topic. If you or someone you know is struggling with sleep during this transition, it would be advisable to work with a health-care provider—ideally, one specializing in menopause and sleep disorders—to create a tailored approach to improving sleep during this transition.

How to Pay Off Your Sleep Debt

If you regularly sleep fewer hours than you need, you will accumulate a *sleep debt*. A small sleep debt may not have noticeable effects, but several nights of insufficient sleep can impair both your body and brain. While sleeping a little longer can help reduce the sleep pressure associated with a few nights of shorter sleep, it won't fully restore the lost balance of sleep stages, like deep NREM and REM sleep, which are essential for recovery and performance. The best approach is to prioritize consistent, sufficient sleep to avoid accumulating sleep debt in the first place.

Naps Can Help, but Watch Out for the Impact on Sleep

Naps can temporarily boost alertness if sleeping longer isn't feasible. A ten- to thirty-minute "power nap" can improve alertness for two to three hours afterward.[233] Getting into bright light after your nap can further enhance the benefits.[234] The performance enhancement associated with a short nap can more than compensate for the time spent napping. Bear in mind that the positive effects of longer naps are more sustained, but sleep inertia—the grogginess we feel upon waking—also increases, which can pose a risk to safety.

If you choose to nap, you should also beware of the potential for sleep interference. Napping allows the brain to clear some *adenosine*, which reduces sleep pressure. However, napping for too long or too close to sleep can reduce sleep pressure too much, making it difficult to get to sleep when needed. Consequently, ensure your nap ends at least eight hours before bed. This should leave time to build up the sleep pressure you'll need to fall asleep again later.

If you often struggle to fall asleep, napping might not be a good idea. Also, if you have never tried napping before, try starting with an early afternoon nap on the weekend to avoid disrupting your sleep during the workweek. Further, napping should not be considered a substitute for sleep.

Some studies have investigated the impact of combining caffeine with napping, affectionately known as a *nappuccino*. This cocktail takes advantage of caffeine requiring about thirty minutes to reach peak levels in our blood plasma. Consuming 200 mg of caffeine (equivalent to a 16-ounce Grande Americano) followed by a twenty-minute nap can provide the alertness-boosting benefits of a nap while reducing the sleep inertia you might feel upon waking.[235,236]

Nonetheless, I would be cautious about using this technique because of the powerful effect of caffeine on sleep.

Breaking the Caffeine Cycle: How Timing Your Last Cup Can Improve Sleep

As I mentioned in chapter 1, caffeine boosts alertness and sharpens cognitive function by blocking adenosine, the neurotransmitter that accumulates during the day and makes us feel drowsy.[33] The half-life of caffeine—how quickly caffeine is processed by the body—can range between one and a half to nine and a half hours but averages around five hours.[237] This means that caffeine's adenosine-blocking, alertness-boosting effects can last four to six hours for most people.

It's also worth noting that oral contraceptives can double the half-life of caffeine.[238] But even with an average half-life, one cup of coffee at any time of day could be enough to disturb your sleep later on.

I often encourage people to try an experiment: Stop caffeine at midday and see if you notice any benefits. Many people find that their sleep improves. Reducing caffeine intake and stopping caffeine earlier can also help some people break a vicious cycle: Consuming caffeine late in the day disrupts sleep, which leads to consuming even more caffeine the next day to combat sleepiness, only to repeat the routine again and again.

Forget the Nightcap: Alcohol Is Not a Sleep Aid

While we're on the topic of substances that can disrupt sleep . . .

Even though many of us may prefer not to read this, the best solution for improving our sleep is to avoid alcohol completely. But if you choose to drink alcohol, better understanding its impact on sleep can at least help you make an informed decision.

It's all too easy to believe that alcohol is a sleep aid. Alcohol reduces the time it takes to fall asleep and can even increase NREM deep sleep initially.[239] This effect creates the impression that alcohol helps sleep, as people feel they fall asleep more quickly and deeply.

However, this perceived benefit comes at the cost of reduced REM sleep—the sleep that is particularly important for learning and memory formation—along with huge disruption to physiological recovery during sleep. As I mentioned in chapter 3, even relatively low doses of alcohol—equivalent to a glass of wine or a beer for a 165-pound (75 kg) adult—can reduce recovery during sleep by almost 10 percent.[129]

It takes approximately one hour to metabolize one unit of alcohol. This means it takes around two hours to metabolize the alcohol in a glass of wine or beer. Consequently, drinking less and stopping earlier may reduce the effects of alcohol on your sleep, even if it doesn't eliminate them. That should not be considered a recommendation to drink at breakfast, though.

Can Wearables Improve Sleep?

As I described in the introduction to this chapter, an increasing number of people are monitoring their sleep with wearable devices.

A recent study investigated the differing ways in which people use and respond to wearable sleep tracking.[240] The researchers identified the following five archetypes:

Critical: Felt sleep tracking harmed their sleep.

Passive: Looked at their sleep data but didn't connect it to their behavior.

Aware: Noticed a connection between their behavior and sleep, sometimes recognizing the need to change.

Reactive: Took some actions to improve their sleep quality based on using a wearable.

Motivated: Actively tried improving sleep based on the metrics.

Over 70 percent of the participants had a neutral or positive experience. Only 6 percent felt that sleep tracking had a negative effect. These data are encouraging because far more people seem to experience benefits from using a wearable than experience harm. However, it's important to recognize that wearable technology may not be appropriate for everyone, particularly if it could increase sleep anxiety.

Orthosomnia—derived from *ortho* (straight or correct) and *somnia* (sleep)—is the dark side of data-driven sleep obsession.[241] It's not a clinical diagnosis such as *insomnia,* which describes difficulties falling asleep or staying asleep. Rather, *orthosomnia* is a societal phenomenon that has emerged as some people become unhealthily obsessed with using sleep data to perfect their sleep. If you sense that this may apply to you, using a sleep-tracking device is probably not a good idea.

How Accurate Are Wearables Anyway?

For those of us who choose to use wearables, it's also worth noting that they may not be as accurate as we've been led to believe.

A recent study examined the accuracy of sixty-two wearable devices relative to gold standard measures.[242] On average, they could identify whether the user was asleep or awake with about 87 percent accuracy. In practice this means that, while these devices cannot measure sleep duration perfectly, they could indicate trends, such as whether you slept generally longer or shorter than usual. They may also be accurate enough to measure sleep and wake timing, for the purposes of estimating social jetlag.

Sleep stage measurement, which often attempts to record time spent in NREM or REM sleep, was much less impressive. Accuracy ranged from 65 to 70 percent. As a result I would be cautious about making decisions or evaluating changes based on wearable sleep staging data. At best the data could be useless. At worst they may have a negative influence.

The Power of Perception: Inaccurate Wearable Data Influences Performance

A study published in the *Journal of Experimental Psychology* revealed that receiving incorrect information about how long people had spent in different sleep stages could have a measurable impact on cognitive performance.[243] Participants were randomly given false feedback about their REM sleep. Those who believed they had more REM sleep performed better, while those told they had less performed worse, even though the feedback did not represent their sleep in reality.

A study among people with insomnia found that participants who received false positive feedback about their sleep quality felt more alert and in a better mood.[244] In contrast, those given negative feedback felt more tired and less alert, regardless of their actual sleep.

More recent research among healthy adults with no sleep disorders underscores the power of suggestion in sleep quality feedback, revealing that even a small adjustment—just 5 percent—to sleep data can have a significantly negative impact.[245] Participants received fabricated sleep feedback resembling the reports from popular wearable devices, showing their sleep quality as better or worse than they had reported. The effects were telling—those given even slightly more negative feedback woke up more frequently during the night, felt less satisfied with their sleep, and reported lower mood, regardless of their actual sleep patterns.

These findings highlight a crucial implication—even minor inaccuracies in wearable sleep data could negatively affect sleep and performance, particularly for people more susceptible to the suggestive power of sleep feedback.

Wearables can be helpful tools for measuring sleep duration and monitoring sleep timing and consistency changes. However, it's crucial to recognize their limitations and accept that sleep tracking is not for everyone.

Also, we all might be better off not knowing how much or how little we've slept, particularly on nights we haven't slept well. For that reason, I often suggest that people who use wearables focus on sleep duration trends over time rather than fixating on the data every morning. I also recommend they consider ignoring their data or leaving the wearable behind during unavoidable periods of sleep disruption, such as during travel.

The Beginner's Mind: Embracing Regenerative Sleep

Whether or not you use a wearable device, it's clear that sleep plays a vital role in health and performance. But we must resist turning sleep into yet another competitive pursuit. By its very nature, sleep eludes conscious control: The harder we try to grasp it, the more it slips through our fingers.

Instead, I encourage you to *consider sleep an experience* rather than something else to work on. Feel free to experiment with ideas that create a welcoming environment for rest with a curious, open shoshin mindset— free from expectations or pressures—so you can discover what truly works for you.

CHAPTER 4 REVIEW

In this chapter we explored the paradox of modern sleep: Despite increased investment in sleep technology and tracking, restful nights remain elusive for many. We examined how different approaches to sleep—from *hyperoptimization* to *sleep denial*—often miss the mark and discovered evidence-based strategies for improving sleep without obsessing over it.

KEY INSIGHTS

SLEEP DURATION AND NEED

- While individual needs vary, adults require between seven to nine hours of sleep.
- The DEC2 "short sleep" gene mutation is extremely rare (0.02 percent).
- Six hours of sleep for two weeks can impair performance, equivalent to two nights without sleep.

ENVIRONMENT MATTERS MOST

Light exposure should be as follows:

- **Day:** Minimum 250 melEDI lux.
- **Evening:** Under 10 melEDI lux.
- **Night:** Under 1 lux.
- Ideal room temperature is between 60°F and 67°F (15.6°C–19.4°C).
- Sound levels should be below 40 decibels.

SLEEP CONSISTENCY IS CRITICAL

- Social jetlag affects 70 percent of people.
- Regular sleep schedules improve health outcomes.
- Consistency and adequate sleep should be prioritized.
- As a backup plan, extra weekend sleep can help offset some weekday deficits.

SLEEP TRACKING CONSIDERATIONS

- Many wearables offer reasonably accurate sleep-wake detection.

- Sleep stage accuracy is much poorer.
- Inaccurate feedback can affect next-day performance.
- Some people develop *orthosomnia* from tracking.

PRACTICAL ACTIONS

1. ASSESS YOUR SLEEP NEED

- Monitor if you can wake up without an alarm.
- Notice if you can nap easily and need stimulants to stay alert during the day.
- Observe your sleep patterns during free days.

2. OPTIMIZE YOUR SLEEP ENVIRONMENT

- Measure and adjust light levels.
- Control room temperature.
- Minimize noise disruption.
- Create near-complete darkness.

3. BUILD SLEEP CONSISTENCY

- Calculate your current social jetlag.
- Work to reduce sleep timing differences.
- Make gradual adjustments (twenty to thirty minutes).
- Try to maintain consistency even on weekends.

Remember This

Sleep is something to be experienced rather than achieved. Focus on creating the right conditions for rest rather than forcing sleep through rigid protocols or excessive tracking.

Looking Ahead

In our next chapter, we'll explore how to increase our energy for everything through regenerative fitness approaches.

CHAPTER 5

REGENERATIVE FITNESS: INCREASE YOUR ENERGY FOR EVERYTHING

More people than ever are exercising. We should be in the best shape of our lives. But we're not.

For most of human history, work was physical. As recently as the 1960s, the majority of jobs required us to expend at least a moderate amount of energy.[246] However, with the rise of knowledge work, productivity shifted from muscles to minds. Today, six in ten people hold office-based roles, and 90 percent of the workday is spent seated.[247,248]

The shift to remote work has only intensified this sedentary trend. Physical activity levels dropped by up to 50 percent as home-based work slashed *incidental activity*: Wandering out to grab lunch, walking to a colleague's desk, or hustling through airports for business trips was traded for video calls.[249]

Knowledge workers are left in a paradoxical situation: They engage in structured exercise, but overall physical activity levels have plummeted.[246,250,251] As a result too many knowledge workers have become *active couch potatoes*—people who complete regular workouts but spend the rest of the day sitting.

Our approach to fitness needs a rethink.

* * *

While most people are familiar with the health benefits of exercise, fewer recognize the risks of sitting for too long. Unfortunately, there is a *dose-response association* (where a greater dose leads to a larger effect) between total sitting time and all-cause mortality—the risk of dying for any reason over a given period.[252] Basically, the longer you sit, the higher the health risk.

Even regular exercise doesn't seem to offset this hazard. Sedentary time is an *independent risk factor*.[253] This means that, even if you exercise regularly, you can't necessarily escape the health risks of sitting for long periods. For example, even if you hit your weekly physical activity target according to the World Health Organization guidelines—at least 150 minutes of moderate-intensity activity, or 75 minutes of vigorous-intensity activity—sitting for more than eight hours each day still significantly increases health risks—particularly in terms of cardiovascular health.[254] For reference, at moderate intensity, breathing is faster, but you're not out of breath. At vigorous intensity, talking is difficult, and you're breathing very hard.

It is possible to offset the risk of sitting for more than eight hours, but only by exercising for at least sixty to seventy-five minutes seven days a week. This is 350 percent greater than the World Health Organization guidelines and more than most knowledge workers can accommodate in their schedules.

The People Who Sit the Most Benefit the Least from Exercise

As if that news weren't bad enough, being sedentary for too long may blunt the health benefits when we finally get the opportunity to exercise. A study published in the *Journal of Applied Physiology* investigated this phenomenon.[255]

An aerobic exercise session such as walking, swimming, or cycling is usually associated with several health benefits, including a reduction in the amount of fat circulating in the bloodstream (lower triglyceride levels), less sugar in the blood (lower blood glucose), and improvements in insulin response (an indicator of how well the body can maintain blood sugar in a healthy range). The researchers carefully controlled the participants' activity levels for several days before measuring these factors.

On the first three days of the study, participants were sedentary for more than thirteen hours, equivalent to taking fewer than four thousand steps per day. On day four, participants either remained sedentary (as a control) or exercised on a treadmill for one hour at moderate intensity.

When the participants exercised for the first time after being sedentary for three days, instead of measuring positive changes, the researchers did not observe any significant variation in these health markers. The researchers concluded that the days of physical inactivity had temporarily made the participants immune to the benefits typically associated with exercise, that is, the people who sat the most benefited the least from exercise.

The results *do not* mean we shouldn't exercise if we've been sedentary. While the benefits may have been blunted in the first session, continuing to exercise regularly while avoiding consecutive days of being sedentary would restore the positive effects. The key message is that we should avoid long periods of sitting, particularly on successive days, where possible.

Sitting for Long Periods May Worsen Mental Health

The dangers of excessive sitting extend beyond physical health, with research linking prolonged sedentary behavior to a 25 percent higher risk of poor mental health outcomes, such as depression.[256] Spending more than three hours per day sedentary, which is typical for many knowledge workers, is also associated with a three to four times greater likelihood of experiencing high levels of psychological stress.[257]

The Risk of Too Much High-Intensity Training

They might be neglecting the dangers of excessive sedentary time, but many knowledge workers have become fixated on high-intensity interval training (HIIT)—a form of exercise featuring alternating bursts of intense effort followed by brief periods of rest or low-intensity activity. The popularity of HIIT has helped it make the American College of Sports Medicine's Worldwide Survey of Fitness Trends for eleven consecutive years.[258]

In many ways this recognition is well deserved. HIIT is versatile and highly effective. One of the most sought-after features for busy knowledge workers is that HIIT is time efficient. For example, some research suggests that HIIT sessions could elicit the same *cardiorespiratory fitness* improvements—a measure of how well your heart, lungs, and muscles work together—in just one-seventh of the time that would be required with lower-intensity training.[259]

The problem is that you can have too much of a good thing. There is an upper limit to the amount of HIIT we can tolerate before things start to go wrong. A study published in the journal *Cell Metabolism* revealed this by exploring the relationship between training volume (the amount of training), training intensity, and the function of *mitochondria*.[260]

Mitochondria are tiny structures inside your cells that act like power plants, producing the energy your body needs to function. They convert nutrients from food into energy that cells can use to power everything from muscle movement to brain activity. HIIT has been shown to improve how well your mitochondria work, making them more efficient at producing energy.

The study's authors recruited average, healthy participants and high-level endurance athletes, prescribing a training program featuring progressively increasing volumes of HIIT. However, rather than seeing continual improvements, once the participants were completing 152 minutes of high-intensity intervals in a week—the equivalent of five HIIT sessions—the researchers noticed some concerning effects.

The participants' glucose regulation—which describes how well they controlled their blood sugar levels—began to be impaired. This suggested that the function of the participants' mitochondria was getting worse rather than better, implying that they had exceeded the beneficial volume of HIIT.

You only need to look at the millions of executives smashing themselves every day of the week in online classes while riding their indoor bikes to see that many knowledge workers are likely exceeding the threshold for benefits, too.

The Risks of Prioritizing Exercise over Sleep

Unfortunately, many people sacrifice sleep to squeeze in their early morning HIIT sessions. Forgoing adequate sleep to make time for any type of exercise isn't advisable. Forcing HIIT sessions into your schedule after several nights of poor sleep might be particularly risky. A recent study underscores this, highlighting that the strain of intense early morning workouts combined with sleep deprivation may do more harm than good.[261]

First, here's a quick lesson on some cardiac physiology: When the heart is damaged, such as during a heart attack, a protein called cardiac troponin

T (cTnT) is released into the bloodstream. Higher cTnT levels can indicate that the heart is under stress or injured.

Researchers measured differences in participants' cTnT levels after completing a HIIT session in two conditions: first, following three nights of sleeping for around eight hours, and second, after sleep was restricted to around four hours a night for three nights.[261]

Following the sleep restriction, the researchers observed a much larger surge of cTnT after the HIIT session. This finding suggests insufficient sleep may lead to an unhealthy cardiac stress response to HIIT.

It's also important to mention that just a single night of sleep deprivation can reduce muscle protein synthesis by 18 percent, increase cortisol levels (a stress hormone) by 21 percent, and decrease testosterone levels in both men and women by 24 percent.[262]

Many high achievers are convinced they get even more fitness benefits by skipping sleep to squeeze in morning workouts. However, these studies strongly suggest that they will benefit less from the sessions if they have not slept enough and may even be causing harm.

A Third Way to Approach Fitness

As we've explored in previous chapters, modern life tends to push us to extremes. Fitness is no exception. In my research and consulting with knowledge workers across the globe, I've witnessed far too many people fall into the trap of emphasizing structured workouts over reducing sedentary time.

I've also seen many cases of the triangular relapse pattern we've explored in previous chapters: People initiate a grueling exercise regime with intense discipline only to find it unsustainable. Motivation wanes, and they return to being relatively inactive, with a few sporadic workouts. This continues for a few more weeks before they dive headfirst back into another punishing program.

It doesn't have to be this way.

There is a more sustainable path that integrates daily movement alongside structured exercise without feeling like you need to push to the limit to get results or beat yourself up if you miss a workout.

Once again this *third* way encourages us to embrace a shoshin mindset by approaching the topic of fitness with an open, curious perspective, appreciating a wide variety of physical activity and exercise types, whether a leisurely stroll or a lung-busting workout.

As a starting point, it's helpful to consider the following five building blocks of fitness:

Move More: Reduce sedentary time.

Move Slow: Lower-intensity aerobic workouts.

Move Fast: High-intensity exercise.

Move Heavy: Resistance training.

Move Together: The benefits of social exercise.

Ideally, we can find a way to incorporate all five into our routine.

Move More: Break Up Sedentary Time

It's easy to fall into the trap of thinking that only structured exercise is associated with health benefits, but this is simply not true.

Any form of physical activity sets off a cascade of internal signals and changes that benefit our body and brain, decreasing the risk of cardiovascular disease and metabolic disorders, reducing anxiety, and improving concentration.

Even tiny *exercise snacks,* such as getting up and moving around for two minutes once every half hour, can reduce the health risks of sitting for long periods.[112] The benefits of moving more extend to mental health, too. Taking a twenty-one-minute walk each day could lower the risk of depression by 18 percent.[263]

What we do while sitting also makes a difference in mental health outcomes. A thirteen-year study involving nearly forty-one thousand participants found that engaging in mentally stimulating activities while sedentary—such as reading or working—significantly reduced the likelihood of experiencing depression compared with spending less time on mentally active tasks and more on passive sedentary activities.[264] Complementary findings show that exchanging just thirty minutes of passive sitting with mentally active behaviors could cut depression risk by 5 percent.[265]

Together, these findings are a powerful reminder of the importance of blending structured exercise with incidental physical activity, such as brief walks between tasks or taking the stairs, as well as keeping our minds active during the time we spend sitting, to offset the downsides of sedentary time.

Moving more also elicits long-term health benefits, such as extending our *health span*—the length of time we will live healthily and disease-free. Reducing sedentary time by three hours could lower our biological age by more than ten months.[266] Walking 9,826 steps daily is associated with a 50 percent risk reduction for developing dementia—a deterioration in cognitive function beyond what might be expected from the usual consequences of biological aging. People who walked at a slightly higher intensity (> 40 steps per minute) cut their risk by 57 percent with just 6,315 steps a day.[267]

Do We All Need to Aim for 10,000 Steps?

All this writing about step counts might get you thinking of the *10,000-step goal*—the popular notion that we should all aim for 10,000 steps daily. But do you know where this supposed rule came from? You might be surprised that it was not based on rigorous research when it was first conceived. Rather, it was a marketing stunt. *Manpo-kei*—translated as "10,000 steps meter"—was introduced in a 1965 sales campaign by a Japanese pedometer manufacturer.

Despite this inauspicious start, the campaign did serve the purpose of getting more people moving. However, it has led to an unhelpful view that we will not experience benefits unless we hit the 10,000-step threshold. This is not true. Wherever you are starting from, health outcomes improve with each additional 1,000 steps taken daily, and we can experience benefits far below the 10,000-step threshold.[268]

While there is no definitive threshold, 7,000 to 8,000 steps per day as a minimum target aligns with public health physical activity guidelines for adults.[269] Aiming for this threshold could also help keep sedentary time below the eight-hour mark, where more significant health risks emerge.[270]

The bottom line is that wherever you're starting from, many of us would benefit from simply moving more.

Move Slow: Build More Cellular Energy Factories

Global life expectancy has doubled since 1900.[271] Most of us want to stay healthy and energetic for as long as possible. One critical physiological capability underpins this aim: our body's ability to regenerate a molecule called *adenosine triphosphate* (ATP).

ATP is a high-energy molecule that, when broken down into smaller components, releases energy that powers everything we do—from moving muscles and digesting meals to solving problems and staying alert. You can think of ATP as the *energy currency of life*.

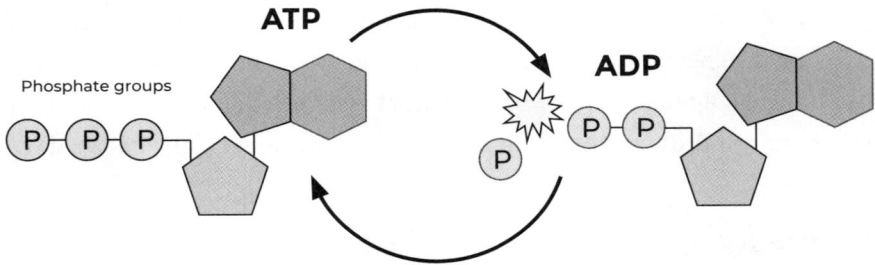

Here's the remarkable part: The average adult requires an amount of ATP equivalent to their body weight every day. Yet our cells hold only a tiny reserve. To keep up with these demands, ATP is constantly recycled within *mitochondria*—the energy factories within our cells—ensuring a seamless supply of energy to sustain life.

When we are healthy, the ATP recycling process within our mitochondria continues without a hitch. However, when it malfunctions, some of the first signs can be seen in the cells that require the most energy.

Age-Related Disorders: A Crisis of Cellular Energy

A growing body of evidence indicates that many age-related disorders—such as type 2 diabetes and Alzheimer's—are related to an energy supply crisis associated with mitochondrial dysfunction. These hypotheses emerged because these conditions are associated with the high-energy tissues of the brain, liver, and heart.[272] As a result, finding ways to maintain the number, health, and function of our mitochondria is critical.

Many people assume that you need to work very hard at high intensity to promote the growth of more mitochondria. However, research indicates that, after adjusting for factors such as training frequency, duration of the training program, and initial fitness, responses are similar between lower-intensity and higher-intensity training.[273]

Integrating regular lower-intensity exercise training—*moving slow*—into your routine can encourage the development of more mitochondria, improve your health and fitness, and potentially ward off energy crises in the future. The following intensity, duration, and frequency principles can help you get started.

Intensity

As I mentioned earlier in this chapter, time-crunched fitness enthusiasts are ramping up the intensity of their sessions, hoping to achieve more in less time. However, lower-intensity training is a potent signal for increasing the number of mitochondria in muscle tissue.[274]

In practice, lower intensity means exercising at up to 70 percent of your *maximum heart rate* if you use a heart rate monitor, where your breathing is faster, but you're not out of breath. For many people, particularly those who are just starting out in their fitness journey, this means a brisk walk rather than a slow run.

You may have heard people quote the "220 minus your age" formula for calculating maximum heart rate, but this is wildly inaccurate. A qualified physiologist or medical professional can determine your maximum heart rate through exercise testing. This figure will enable you to calculate your 70 percent threshold. Using a heart rate monitor can provide real-time feedback to ensure you stay below this target.

Alternatively, you could base your effort on *perceived exertion* (how hard you feel you are working). Our perception is a surprisingly accurate measure of exercise intensity that continues to be used by many of the world's top endurance athletes despite the availability of sophisticated technological measurement systems. On a scale from 0 to 10, where 0 represented no effort and 10 was maximal, these aerobic sessions usually fall in the 4 to 6 range, representing a comfortable and sustainable effort. As a rule of thumb, you should be able to speak in a complete sentence at this intensity.

Duration

The length of aerobic workouts can vary based on fitness level and training goals. For instance, a thirty-minute continuous jog might be appropriate for beginners, while more advanced athletes might go for runs lasting ninety minutes to two hours or even longer.

A good starting point is to work toward completing at least 150 minutes of lower-intensity aerobic activity each week. This could be based on structured exercise—such as several running, swimming, or cycling sessions—but it doesn't have to be. Walking or cycling from place to place is often more than adequate.

While this lower-intensity exercise may not feel particularly effortful or effective, repeated muscle contractions over extended periods provide a powerful stimulus for gene expression, which increases the number of mitochondria.[275] Many fitness enthusiasts miss out on this valuable low-intensity training because they're convinced that no pain means no gain. They are wrong.

Low-intensity exercise also offers impressive benefits for mental health. Researchers analyzed the results of multiple well-controlled studies that compared exercise to antidepressants. Four months of exercising for 150 minutes per week at moderate intensity— equivalent to a brisk walk for most people—had a similar impact on depression as taking an antidepressant.[276] That is not to say exercise should replace prescribed medication, though. Mental health is incredibly complex, and the most effective treatments should be discussed with an appropriately qualified professional. However, it's encouraging to see research indicating that physical activity can have a clinically meaningful impact on mental health.

Frequency

Ideally, we would integrate aerobic exercise sessions throughout our week. However, many people struggle to find time. I'm often asked whether cramming your aerobic exercise into the weekend in one or two longer sessions offers the same benefits as shorter, more frequent sessions. One study investigated this question by comparing the effects of squeezing exercise into one or two days versus dividing it over three to five days.[277]

Based on data from approximately 350,000 adults, the analyses revealed that both approaches are similarly effective in improving health outcomes. A more recent study confirmed this finding based on data from academically validated wearables.[278] Compressing activity in one to two days was associated with a similar reduction in cardiovascular disease risk compared with more frequent exercisers. The benefits of exercise for brain health, such as reducing the risk of cognitive impairment and dementia, also remain even if people do all their exercise in a couple of days rather than divided over the week.[279]

Great news for the weekend warriors.

These studies' complementary and supportive findings are encouraging, and the implications are clear: Aerobic exercise will likely be beneficial any day of the week. So rather than getting too fixated on thresholds, durations, and frequencies, I encourage you to focus on getting started, even if you only manage a few minutes of activity.

Move Fast: Introducing VO$_2$ Max—the Vital Sign You Didn't Know You Needed

Have you watched a world-class endurance sports event such as the Tour de France or Olympic cross-country skiing? If you have, I imagine you have heard commentators talking about *VO$_2$ max*.

VO$_2$ max describes the maximum rate at which our body can take up and use oxygen during strenuous exercise. It's usually expressed as the amount of oxygen someone can take up and use measured in milliliters relative to their body mass in kilograms per minute (mL/kg/min). Physiologists assess VO_2 max by asking people to exert themselves, often by running or cycling, at progressively faster speeds, usually while monitoring their breathing rates and the changing properties of the air they breathe in and out.

I'm continually amazed by the physiology of world-class performers. A group of researchers from Norway published a paper describing VO_2 max benchmark values across endurance sports in the Winter Olympics.[280] The study suggests that to win a medal in cross-country skiing, a male competitor requires a VO_2 max of around 84 mL/kg/min and a female athlete 72 mL/kg/min. To put that in perspective, a thirty- to fifty-year-old nonathlete would be considered to be in good physical condition if they can achieve 50 percent of these VO_2 max values: around 43 mL/kg/min in men or 34 mL/kg/min in women.[281]

VO₂ Max Matters for Elite Athletes and Average Joes

VO_2 max is about much more than physical performance, though. This value represents the outcome of many critical physiological systems working together. Such is its importance; some clinicians argue that VO_2 max should be considered a vital sign alongside measures such as blood pressure.[282]

A meta-analysis of thirty-seven studies involving two million participants adds weight to this claim. Increasing VO_2 max by just 3.5 ml/kg/min could cut all-cause mortality by 11 percent.[283] Having a VO_2 max in the top third reduces all-cause mortality by 45 percent compared with those in the bottom third.

VO_2 max may even predict when we can no longer live independently in later life.[284] For instance, someone in the bottom tenth percentile for VO_2 max could expect to begin relying on other people because of reduced physical capacity in their early seventies. In contrast, someone in the top ninetieth percentile could expect to remain independent for the rest of their life. The more you can increase your VO_2 max while you are younger, the better you can maintain it as you age and the longer and healthier your life is likely to be.

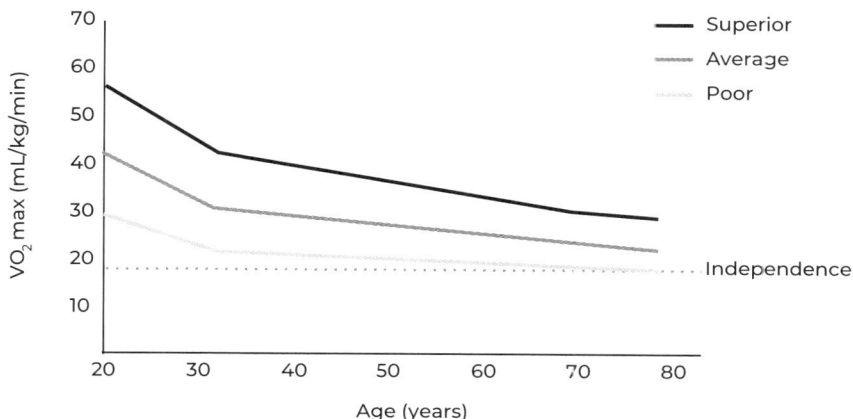

Adapted based on Gries, K. J. et al. (2018) 'Cardiovascular and skeletal muscle health with lifelong exercise.'

How Do You Compare?

Several methods are available if you're curious to measure your VO_2 max. The most accurate requires a physical effort that is both long and intense enough to tax the aerobic energy system fully. This typically involves visiting a laboratory to endure a graded exercise test where exercise intensity is progressively increased. There are also several ways to estimate VO_2 max, which don't require a trip to the lab. Recent studies suggest that some wearables can estimate VO_2 max with reasonable accuracy.[285,286,287]

Once you've measured or estimated your VO_2 max, many people's next question is how they compare with others and what value represents a good level. Several studies have examined this question. I've summarized the results of one study in the tables below.[281] All values are expressed in mL/kg/min.

VO₂ Standards for Women

AGE	LOW	BELOW AVERAGE	ABOVE AVERAGE	HIGH	ELITE
18-19	<35.0	35.0-38.5	38.9-45.2	45.5-52.2	≥52.5
20-29	<28.0	28.0-34.6	35.0-39.9	40.3-49.7	≥50.0
30-39	<27.0	27.0-32.6	32.9-37.8	38.2-47.6	≥48.0
40-49	<25.9	25.9-31.2	31.5-36.1	36.4-46.2	≥46.6
50-59	<24.5	24.5-28.0	28.4-34.6	35.0-45.2	≥45.5
60-69	<21.0	21.0-24.2	24.5-29.4	29.8-38.5	≥38.9
70-79	<17.5	17.5-20.7	21.0-24.2	24.5-34.6	≥35.0
≥80	<15.4	15.4-18.9	19.3-21.7	22.1-29.1	≥29.4

VO₂ Standards for Men

AGE	LOW	BELOW AVERAGE	ABOVE AVERAGE	HIGH	ELITE
18-19	<37.8	37.8-45.2	45.5-48.7	49.0-56.7	≥57.1
20-29	<36.1	36.1-41.6	42.0-47.6	48.0-54.6	≥55.0
30-39	<35.0	35.0-38.9	39.2-45.2	45.5-52.2	≥52.5
40-49	<34.3	34.3-38.2	38.5-43.4	43.8-51.1	≥51.5
50-59	<28.7	28.7-34.6	35.0-39.6	39.9-48.7	≥49.0
60-69	<24.5	24.5-29.4	29.8-34.6	35.0-45.2	≥45.5
70-79	<21.0	21.0-24.2	24.5-29.4	29.8-39.9	≥40.3
≥80	<17.9	17.9-21.7	22.1-25.2	25.6-34.6	≥35.0

So if having a higher VO₂ max is so great, the obvious question is, how can we maintain and improve it?

How to Improve Your VO$_2$ Max

The best way to ensure you end up with a world-class VO$_2$ max is to choose your parents wisely—25 to 50 percent of the difference in VO$_2$ max among individuals is inherited.[288] But even if we don't begin with elite potential, we can all improve our VO$_2$ max. Some people may even be able to achieve improvements over 90 percent.[289]

Also, declines in VO$_2$ max as we age are inevitable to some extent, but not as much as we may think. Changes in training volume explain more than 50 percent of the reductions in VO$_2$ max seen in athletes as they age.[290] The implication is that we may be able to offset much of this decline by continuing to exercise regularly as we get older.

Further, even if VO$_2$ max has decreased through reduced training, it can bounce back quickly. VO$_2$ max increases of 9 to 13 percent were observed after eight weeks of HIIT in men and women aged from twenty to more than seventy, following a return to training after time off. The implication is that it's never too late to start improving your VO$_2$ max or to start again.

Low- and moderate-intensity aerobic exercise, as described in the *Move Slow* section, is an effective way to improve VO$_2$ max. However, HIIT is very time efficient.[273,291] With the caveat that we can do too much HIIT (as I mentioned earlier) and providing you don't have any underlying health conditions to hold you back, you can integrate HIIT into your routine based on the following considerations:

Intensity

HIIT sessions involve interspersing intense efforts with periods of recovery. The intense efforts are generally performed at 85 to 95 percent of the maximum heart rate, while recovery periods are usually around 40 to 50 percent. The target intensity is a function of the duration of each intense interval. Shorter intervals—which could be as brief as twenty seconds—can be performed at higher intensity. In comparison, longer intervals—which could last for up to eight minutes—are performed at relatively lower intensity.

HIIT sessions are effective across various work-recovery ratios, so feel free to experiment. Common formats include thirty seconds of intense effort followed by thirty seconds of low-intensity recovery at the shorter end. At the longer end, four minutes of work followed by four minutes of rest is typical. A personal favorite of mine features a warm-up followed by five minutes at 85 percent of my maximum effort and then five minutes of low-intensity recovery repeated five times. However, I worked to the point that I could tolerate and benefit from this format over several years.

As I mentioned, you could use a heart rate monitor to ensure you work at the appropriate intensity. However, it's important to note that your heart rate will not immediately spike as soon as you begin an intense interval. The idea is that you work hard to reach the target intensity range during each interval.

As I suggested in the *Move Slow* section, you don't need to use a heart rate monitor or other measurement technology if you'd prefer not to. You can gauge intensity using perceived exertion. On a scale of 1 to 10 (with 10 being the maximum effort), the intense portions of HIIT intervals often fall in the 8 to 10 range, with recovery periods at a 2 or 3.

Duration

A typical HIIT session—including warm-up, intervals, and cooldown—might last between twenty and sixty minutes, but don't let lack of time hold you back. In one study, researchers prescribed ten-minute sessions featuring a series of ten- to twenty-second all-out sprints. Participants completed these sessions three times per week for six weeks, resulting in 12 to 15 percent improvements in VO_2 max.[292]

In another study, researchers investigated the effects of brief, intense *exercise snacks* on VO_2 max.[293] Three times each day, three days each week, for six weeks, a group of relatively sedentary participants completed a stair-climbing exercise. This involved climbing three flights of stairs (equivalent to sixty steps) at hard intensity, repeated three times. This routine equated to three sets of twenty seconds of hard effort as they quickly climbed the stairs, followed by two minutes of recovery as they walked slowly back down. The daily sessions amounted to ten minutes of total exercise time on each of the three days. Despite this low training volume, the participants experienced a 5 percent increase in VO_2 max.

Frequency

As I described earlier in this chapter, there is a threshold beyond which HIIT may no longer be beneficial, but this is not the only downside of doing HIIT too often. When people try to complete HIIT sessions too frequently, they cannot recover adequately and struggle to hit the high intensities that characterize a true HIIT session. As a result their HIIT sessions become moderate-intensity sessions, often without them realizing it. These sessions are fatiguing without eliciting the VO_2 max–boosting benefits of well-executed HIIT. Falling into this middle zone often results in a plateau in fitness improvements and an enduring sense of tiredness.

We actually don't need much HIIT in our routine for it to be effective. Even world-class athletes use HIIT very sparingly. To use a culinary metaphor, HIIT should be the carefully applied seasoning in a training program, not the main course. As a rule of thumb, one properly executed HIIT session per week is likely sufficient for most people.

The Benefits of HIIT Extend Far Beyond VO_2 Max

In addition to increasing VO_2 max, HIIT is associated with a wide range of additional health benefits. For example, a twelve-minute high-intensity *exercise snack* thirty minutes before mealtimes could reduce twenty-four-hour mean blood glucose concentration, an indication of metabolic health, more than a continuous exercise session twice as long.[294]

A recent study investigated the benefits of *vigorous intermittent lifestyle physical activity* (VILPA), a variation of HIIT. Think of VILPA as a high-intensity exercise snack where everyday activities, such as running up the stairs or through an airport, are turned into an opportunity to boost health.[295] Researchers observed a striking pattern over nearly seven years of data: Engaging in just three one- to two-minute VILPA bursts each day was associated with a 38 to 40 percent reduction in all-cause and cancer mortality risk and a 48 to 49 percent reduction in cardiovascular disease mortality risk. Similar results were found in exercisers and nonexercisers, pointing to VILPA's benefits for a broad range of people.

High-intensity exercise can also reduce negative stress and provide a mood boost.[296] Recent research found that HIIT significantly improves memory and brain function in older adults.[297] Changes in specific blood markers also suggest HIIT may help protect against cognitive decline in aging.[297]

If you have no underlying health conditions preventing you, you can try integrating HIIT into your exercise routine. However, people who have done little to no exercise or who are unfamiliar with high-intensity training should approach HIIT with care under the instruction of an appropriately qualified professional.

Move Heavy: Muscles Are About More than Looks

Muscular physiques are increasingly *en vogue,* but the reasons for building and maintaining muscle mass extend far beyond vanity.

After age thirty, we can begin to lose muscle at a rate of around 3 to 5 percent per decade. After turning fifty, muscle mass begins to decrease at a rate of 1 to 2 percent per year, and muscle strength declines at 1.5 to 5 percent per year.[298] Consequently, if we don't actively build and maintain muscle in later life, we could end up with an adult-size skeleton with the muscle mass of a child.

Low muscle mass is associated with an increased risk of many adverse health outcomes. In contrast, building and maintaining muscle has many benefits, including improving metabolic health and reducing the risk of cardiovascular heart disease.[299] It's perhaps no surprise that being in the top 25 percent of muscle mass for your age group is a significant positive predictor of longevity.[300] Peak muscle power is also a significant predictor of how well we'll be able to move and function in later life.[301]

It can also be helpful to think about muscle mass and strength in terms of how it can benefit everyday life. Instead of imagining pumping iron into your old age, think about being in your seventies and still able to lift your hand luggage into an overhead compartment on a plane without assistance, carry your shopping bags, or have the strength to stop yourself from falling if you were to trip. Contrary to popular belief, falling is not a normal part of aging—it's often related, to a large degree, to preventable declines in muscle mass and strength. We can significantly offset the risk of falls, remain independent, and improve our quality of life by maintaining and building our muscle size and strength.

* * *

Resistance exercise, sometimes called weight training, is an effective way to increase muscle mass and strength, but you don't necessarily need weights. Bodyweight exercises and resistance bands, which you can use at home, can also work well as you get started.

Guidelines for physical activity highlight the importance of engaging in strength and resistance exercises at least two days per week.[254] However, it's essential to be aware that there is a risk of injury if you are not familiar with the movement patterns of resistance training exercises. I strongly recommend working with a qualified coach or fitness trainer before integrating resistance exercise into your routine.

The ideal time to build and reach peak muscle mass is before the age of fifty. But don't despair; improvements are possible at almost every stage of life. Studies have demonstrated that ninety-year-olds can improve their muscle strength with the appropriate training.[302] Providing no underlying health issues are holding you back, today is the best time to begin.

Move Together

Ever noticed that exercise feels easier in a group? Data from Strava, the world's largest social network for athletes, reveals a consistent trend: When we work out with others, we tend to go further and stay active longer.[303]

For example, runners in pairs ran for 21 percent longer and 15 percent further than if they were running solo. Cyclists averaged 29 km per ride alone, while those in groups averaged 49 km. In January, when the weather is often at its worst in the northern hemisphere, cyclists and runners who exercised with others recorded 87 percent and 78 percent more active time than their solo peers. Why could this be?

Research reveals that social support significantly influences how we perceive challenges.[111,304] For example, when accompanied by a friend, participants perceived hills to be less steep than alone. Intriguingly, even thinking about a supportive person was associated with a benefit. Wherever you are in your fitness journey, I encourage you to find some people to join you.

That said, we should also be careful not to judge our exercise habits relative to others. If you use social media or platforms such as Strava, it can seem like every other person is preparing for a marathon, triathlon, or getting in 10,000 steps before breakfast. Evidence indicates that comparing our activity levels with others could worsen mental well-being. For example, participants in a recent study completed a survey to assess their actual sedentary time relative to their perception of how sedentary they were compared with others.[305] When people perceived themselves as more sedentary than others, they felt more stressed.

These findings are an important reminder that everyone's path is different. Some days will be more or less active than others. Celebrate your progress and achievements rather than compare yourself with others.

In Closing

Fitness is a vast topic. Each of us responds to different types of exercise in subtly different ways. However, the fundamentals remain, and the simple actions often make the biggest difference. We should seek to avoid the traps of overemphasizing structured exercise while ignoring sedentary lifestyles or overdosing on HIIT while ignoring the benefits of low-intensity, slow sessions. And we'll all benefit from lifting some heavy things a couple of times a week. But if I were only to leave you with one principle to help you find your *third way*, it would be this: When it comes to movement and exercise, something is better than nothing.

CHAPTER 5 REVIEW

In this chapter we explored the paradox of modern fitness: Despite record gym membership numbers, overall physical activity has plummeted. We examined how knowledge workers have become *active couch potatoes* and discovered that mixing different types of movement—from reducing sedentary time to engaging in high-intensity training—is crucial for both health and performance.

KEY INSIGHTS

THE SEDENTARY CRISIS

- Physical activity levels dropped up to 50 percent with remote work.
- Sitting over eight hours daily increases health risks significantly.
- Even regular exercise doesn't fully offset prolonged sitting.
- Extended sedentary time can make exercise less effective.

BUILDING BLOCKS OF FITNESS

- **Move More:** Break up sedentary time.
- **Move Slow:** Lower-intensity aerobic workouts.
- **Move Fast:** High-intensity exercise.
- **Move Heavy:** Resistance training.
- **Move Together:** Social exercise benefits.

VO$_2$ MAX IMPORTANCE

- Could be considered a vital sign alongside blood pressure.
- 3.5 mL/kg/min increase cuts mortality risk by 11 percent.
- Can predict independence in later life.
- Improvements possible at any age.

HIIT CONSIDERATIONS

- Time efficient but has upper limits.
- More than 152 minutes weekly can be counterproductive.
- Sleep deprivation may increase cardiac stress during HIIT.
- One session per week is sufficient for most people.

PRACTICAL ACTIONS

1. BREAK UP SEDENTARY TIME

- Take two-minute movement breaks every thirty minutes.
- Aim for a daily minimum of 7,000 to 8,000 steps.
- Include movement in daily activities.
- Build in regular standing breaks.

2. BALANCE EXERCISE TYPES

- Include low-intensity aerobic activity.
- Add one weekly HIIT session.
- Incorporate resistance training twice weekly.
- Exercise with others when possible.

3. MONITOR EXERCISE INTENSITY

- Can use wearables, but perceived exertion scales are very effective.
- Keep most aerobic exercise conversational.
- Ensure adequate recovery between intense sessions.
- Listen to your body's signals.

Remember This

When it comes to movement and exercise, something is better than nothing. Focus on consistency over intensity and remember that all forms of movement contribute to health and fitness.

Looking Ahead

In our next chapter, we'll explore how to cut through the noise of nutrition advice and find sustainable approaches to eating.

CHAPTER 6

REGENERATIVE NUTRITION: CUTTING THROUGH THE NOISE

Why is nutrition advice so contradictory? And why does it seem to change all the time?

You will struggle to find consensus when it comes to diets, but you'll have no difficulty finding evangelists for almost every imaginable way of eating with convincing-sounding arguments for why you should eat that way, too. *Keto Crusaders* are convinced high fat, low carb is the key to metabolic mastery. *Vegan Zealots* are plant based in everything. *Intermittent Fasting* fanatics believe less is more when it comes to meal frequency. Don't get me started on the *Carnivore Diet,* where it's all meat all the time.

If finding the right diet weren't hard enough, nutritional advice seems to be in constant flux. What was once considered a dietary truth can suddenly be turned on its head, leaving many people confused about what they should be eating. And if they somehow manage to sift through the contradictory advice and discover a diet that works for them, finding the time and energy to stick to it is another story. Eating well can feel like another task in an already overloaded to-do list.

As a result, many people fall into the familiar *triangular relapse pattern* we've explored in previous chapters. First comes the initial enthusiasm and commitment to hyperoptimization as they meticulously count macros, prepare meals, and avoid all processed foods for a few weeks. Then the setbacks hit. Pressures of work, tight deadlines, endless meetings, and late-night emails mean their healthy lunch turns into a quick bite between calls, and the evening meal becomes whatever's most convenient.

Too often, people feel guilty, like they have failed, and *quiet quit,* falling back into unhealthy habits, only to restart the hyperoptimization process once they summon the willpower and motivation again.

But the problem is not a lack of willpower or motivation; it's the myth that there is a single perfect way to eat and that we must follow it unfalteringly. However, that nuance is often lost in the cacophony of dietary advice from influencers, diet gurus, and the media.

Why Is There So Much Conflicting Advice?

One key reason dietary advice often feels contradictory is that nutrition research is incredibly challenging. Scientists typically aim to isolate variables to clarify relationships, such as the impact of a specific nutrient on health. Yet in real life we don't consume isolated nutrients—we eat meals with multiple ingredients that interact in complex ways.

Consider a simple salad: Its blend of vitamins, minerals, fiber, fats, and other compounds interacts in ways that affect how each nutrient is digested and absorbed. This complexity grows when you factor in individual differences—two people might eat the same meal, yet their bodies can respond differently because of variations in metabolism, gut microbiome, genetics, and lifestyle elements such as sleep, exercise, and stress levels.

When we take into account the countless combinations of foods and nutrients we consume daily, along with the unique responses each person may have, it becomes clearer why nutrition research is far from straightforward.

Why High-Quality Nutrition Research Is So Challenging

Scientists also face a tough choice when designing their studies. Controlled laboratory studies—where researchers dictate exactly what participants eat and monitor every meal—offer precise data and can reduce the influence of some lifestyle factors, but this level of oversight and regulation is only feasible for short periods. It's unrealistic to lock people in a lab for months or years. On the other hand, real-world studies allow researchers to observe how people eat in their natural environments over longer periods, but they come with significant trade-offs. Participants may not follow the diet as prescribed or forget to report meals accurately, making it harder to draw clear conclusions.

This tug-of-war between control and practicality is one reason nutritional findings can appear contradictory. What works in a tightly controlled setting may not translate to the chaos of everyday life, and what seems effective for one group of people may not hold for another. Scientists are constantly refining their understanding as they try to untangle the web of interactions that influence how food affects our bodies. While guidelines emerge from the best available evidence, they're often just pieces of a larger, more complex puzzle.

* * *

So where does this leave us? It's impossible to cover every aspect of nutrition in a single book, let alone one chapter. The solution lies, once again, in finding a *third way* that avoids extremes and breaks unhelpful cycles by adopting a more flexible approach to eating. The first step in finding this way is to cut through some of the noise surrounding nutrition.

This chapter distills the current evidence and expert consensus into foundational principles and key ideas that you can use to evaluate the nutrition content you come across and make more intuitive, evidence-based eating decisions that support health, well-being, and performance.

I encourage you to approach this chapter—and the topic of nutrition more broadly—with a shoshin beginner's mindset, marked by openness and curiosity. Our understanding of nutrition continues to evolve, so staying open to new insights is key.

Is Processed Food Bad? It Depends.

A simple, powerful, healthy eating principle is to choose minimally processed foods whenever possible, but it's important to recognize that food processing is not always harmful. The NOVA food classification system offers a clear breakdown of four levels of processing, helping us distinguish between foods that retain their natural benefits and those that may have lost them along the way.[306]

Unprocessed/minimally processed foods: These natural foods have undergone simple physical changes without any chemical processing. Examples include removing inedible parts, drying, crushing, or grinding. Think fresh fruits, vegetables, meats, ground coffee, mashed potatoes, and nut butters—provided no salt, sugar, oils, or other ingredients are added.

Processed culinary ingredients: These are extracted directly from unprocessed or minimally processed foods or sourced from nature through methods such as pressing or refining. Examples include oils, salt, and spices.

Processed foods: These are products created by combining *processed ingredients* with *unprocessed* or *minimally processed* foods. Examples include canned vegetables and fruits preserved in syrup.

Ultraprocessed foods: These are products primarily made from food extracts combined with additives such as flavor enhancers and preservatives. Examples include soft drinks, packaged snacks, and reconstituted meat products.

Imagine the NOVA classification as a hierarchy where ultraprocessed foods are the most problematic. Ideally, our diets would favor unprocessed and minimally processed foods with a few whole food–based processed culinary ingredients. Regrettably, recent decades have seen a massive increase in the consumption of ultraprocessed foods, mainly because they are cheap, have a long shelf life, and are quick and easy to eat.

Further, many ultraprocessed foods feature a blend of sugar, salt, and fat designed to hit our *bliss point*—a Goldilocks zone for sweetness, saltiness, and richness that makes foods hyperpalatable, hijacking our appetite regulation and encouraging overeating.[307] Ultraprocessing can also degrade nutrients and produce harmful compounds, while additives and packaging chemicals have been linked to inflammation and hormonal disruption.[308,309] This combination of appetite dysregulation and low nutrient density means that high consumption of ultraprocessed food often leaves people overfed and undernourished.

Ultraprocessed Foods: Gut Health's Silent Saboteur

On top of that, ultraprocessed foods may harm our *gut* microbiome—a collection of trillions of tiny organisms that live in our digestive system and play a crucial role in keeping us healthy. Most evidence linking ultraprocessed foods to gut disease comes from observational studies, which makes establishing a direct causal relationship challenging. However, mounting evidence suggests a troubling connection between these foods and adverse health outcomes.[308]

These findings may relate to the fact that ultraprocessing often strips away *fiber*—a type of indigestible carbohydrate naturally occurring in plants—from its whole food source. Take flour, for example. Whole wheat flour contains entire grains, which include three components: the *bran* (rich in fiber), the *germ* (containing vitamins and minerals such as B vitamins and iron), and the *endosperm* (which is mostly starch—a complex carbohydrate found in many plants). To make white flour, the fiber-rich bran and the vitamin- and mineral-packed germ are removed. The result is a low-fiber, nutrient-depleted product that offers fewer health benefits. Its only advantages are a lower cost and a longer shelf life.

Cheap Ultraprocessed Foods May Carry a High Health Cost

The fiber deficit in diets heavy in ultraprocessed foods poses a serious issue. In a well-balanced gut, good bacteria ferment fiber, creating an environment that favors beneficial microbes, reduces inflammation, strengthens the gut lining, and supports healthy digestion. Without enough fiber, this balance falters, fostering conditions that allow harmful bacteria to thrive, potentially degrading gut health and contributing to broader health risks.

For example, higher ultraprocessed food consumption has been associated with a greater risk of inflammatory bowel disease, irritable bowel syndrome, and even colorectal cancer.[308] A review of studies involving nearly 190,000 participants, ranging from children to older adults, found that higher consumption of ultraprocessed foods was associated with a 26 percent higher risk of obesity.[310,311] Eating more ultraprocessed food is associated with a greater risk of high blood pressure, cardiovascular diseases, diabetes, and *all-cause mortality*.[309,312,313,314]

Alongside that, a recent study examined changes in *cognition*—how our brain gathers, processes, stores, and uses information—associated with ultraprocessed food consumption.[315] For all participants—except those in the bottom 25 percent who consumed the least—eating ultraprocessed foods was linked to a 28 percent faster rate of overall cognitive decline.

This doesn't mean we can't enjoy the occasional doughnut—these negative effects usually result from high consumption—but limiting our ultraprocessed food intake would likely benefit us all.

Practical Tips for a Whole-Food, High-Fiber Plate

To put these insights into practice, bias your diet toward whole food sources that were running, swimming, flying, or growing, with as few processing steps as possible before they make it to your plate. Think grilled chicken over chicken nuggets or steel-cut oats rather than flavored instant oatmeal.

A fiber-rich diet is also key. Aim for two servings of fruits or vegetables with each meal and eat a rainbow of colors throughout the week. This means incorporating a range of vibrant hues—such as red, green, yellow, orange, and purple—from a variety of fresh produce. For example, you could start the day with blueberries and an apple, enjoy a leafy green salad with red and yellow bell peppers for lunch, and have carrots and eggplant for dinner. This diversity supports gut health and ensures a broad array of nutrients.

Macronutrients: Understanding the Building Blocks of Our Diet

One of the simplest ways to start thinking about our food is as a collection of *macronutrients*. A macronutrient is a type of nutrient that your body needs in large amounts to function properly. There are three main macronutrients: carbohydrates, fats, and protein. Each provides your body with energy (measured in calories) and plays specific roles in keeping you healthy.

Carbohydrates provide quick energy, especially for your brain and muscles.

Proteins help build and repair muscles and tissues.

Fats give long-lasting energy and help with essential functions such as absorbing specific vitamins, cell structure, and hormone production, to name just a few.

In addition to having different roles, each macronutrient has a different *energy density*. Carbohydrates and protein each provide four calories per gram. Fat is the most energy dense, providing nine calories per gram.

Incidentally, alcohol, while not a macronutrient, is often considered in energy calculations. It provides seven calories per gram. If someone had told me that before I went to university, I could have avoided gaining a few pounds.

In short, macronutrients are the building blocks of your diet, giving you energy and helping your body run smoothly.

The Carbohydrate Controversy: Separating Fact from Fiction

Unfortunately, some people have made it a mission to demonize particular macronutrients. For instance, restricting carbohydrates has become increasingly popular in recent years, the most extreme expression being the ketogenic diet, where carbohydrate intake is limited to fewer than fifty grams per day.[316]

More moderate low-carb diets are also prevalent, but regardless of the exact quantities, advocates often promote the approach based on the notion that eating carbohydrates spikes blood sugar and insulin levels. Gary Taubes—a journalist and prominent advocate for low-carbohydrate diets—heavily promoted this theory, including in his best-selling book *Why We Get Fat.*[317]

Taubes became well known for challenging the *calories in, calories out model*. He suggested carbohydrate restriction—rather than calorie counting—was the key to weight loss and health improvement. His argument was based on the carbohydrate-insulin model of obesity, which contends that obesity is driven by carbohydrate consumption and the associated insulin response rather than excess calorie intake.

If you remember chapter 1, you might question whether this could be an example of *biological plausibility bias*—where we assume that a claim is true and that there is a cause-and-effect relationship simply because there is a logical-sounding biological link.

To his credit, Taubes wanted to provide more rigorous scientific evidence to support his hypothesis, so in 2012 he cofounded the Nutrition Science Initiative, with a particular focus on testing his theories.

One of their most prominent studies was led by Dr. Kevin Hall, a scientist specializing in the regulation of body weight and metabolism. He placed participants in tightly controlled environments and compared low-carbohydrate, high-fat diets with high-carbohydrate, low-fat diets while keeping protein levels consistent.

The results showed that although participants on the low-carbohydrate diet initially lost more weight in the first few weeks, this advantage diminished over time, and both groups experienced similar overall fat loss.[318] Additionally, the study didn't find the dramatic metabolic advantages of low-carb diets that the carbohydrate-insulin model predicted.[319] Ultimately, Dr. Hall concluded that the carbohydrate-insulin model of obesity was "difficult to reconcile with current evidence."[320]

While Taubes had expected the research to solidify his views, the answers were less clear-cut than he might have hoped.

Processing Is the Real Enemy in the Carbohydrate Story

More recent research has continued to test the model. However, rather than carbohydrates being inherently harmful, food manufacturers' *industrial processing* of carbohydrates appears to be the culprit.[321] This processing and stripping away of fiber reduces the *nutrient density* and can elicit potentially harmful effects, such as large, rapid spikes in blood glucose levels. Consequently, for most people, the solution is not to avoid carbohydrates but to limit consumption from highly processed sources. For example, eating a potato is likely a much healthier choice than a potato chip.

Further, you could consider how carbohydrate sources are combined and ordered alongside other foods. For example, research in people with type 2 diabetes indicates that consuming vegetables and proteins before carbohydrates may slow glucose absorption into the bloodstream and reduce spikes.[322] In practice this could mean eating a tuna salad before you tuck into some air-fried baby potatoes.

We can also use exercise to reduce the size of spikes and fluctuations in blood sugar after eating, with potential benefits for cardiovascular and metabolic health.[323, 324, 325] For generations, Italians have enjoyed *passeggiata*—a short stroll after meals. A recent study provided a new perspective on this tradition. Just thirty minutes of walking fifteen minutes after finishing a meal significantly reduced blood sugar concentrations in healthy people.[325]

In other instances carbohydrates' ability to quickly increase blood glucose is ideal. If you need energy quickly—such as for a hard workout—increasing carbohydrate intake before, during, and after the workout, even from more processed sources, will likely improve your performance and help you recover faster.

When it comes to carbohydrates, understanding the context is key. However, as a general rule of thumb, minimally processed carbohydrate sources—such as sweet potatoes, squash, fruits, and sprouted grain breads (where the whole grains have been allowed to germinate, or sprout, before being milled to enhance the grain's nutrient profile)—can make up a healthy and beneficial portion of a nutritious diet.

Protein Is Critical for Muscle Maintenance and Appetite Regulation

In the previous chapter, I mentioned how building and maintaining muscle is critical for increasing our *health span*—the length of time we will live healthily and free from disease.

Protein is essential to this muscle-building and maintaining process. Unfortunately, as we age, we become more resistant to the anabolic, muscle-building properties of the protein in our diets.[326,327] Consequently, evidence makes it clear that many of us would benefit from consuming at least 1.2 to 1.4 grams of protein per kilogram of body weight daily.[328,329] This translates to approximately 0.54 to 0.64 grams per pound of body weight. So a 165-pound (75 kg) person would need approximately 90 to 105 grams of protein daily, according to this recommendation. You may notice that this amount is substantially higher than the recommended daily allowance (RDA) set by US food agencies and the World Health Organization, which recommend just 0.8 grams of protein per kilogram of body weight per day.[330] This is because these RDA values are designed to cover basic nutritional needs and prevent deficiencies at a population level, not to improve health or performance.

Protein consumption also reduces *ghrelin*—an appetite-stimulating hormone—more than other macronutrients. This makes protein more satiating than carbohydrates or fat, helping you feel fuller for longer, potentially supporting weight loss (or maintaining a healthy weight) by reducing the likelihood of overeating.[331]

Protein Myths: What Science Really Says

Despite these well-documented benefits, protein is still associated with a lot of misinformation and misunderstanding—mainly concerning fears about the potential health risks of higher protein diets or protein supplementation on kidney function. The theory that high protein intake harms kidney function, even in healthy people, is more than forty years old, but it was never supported by good evidence.

A recent comprehensive systematic review and meta-analysis of high-quality studies examined the impact of higher protein diets on kidney function in healthy adults.[332] The average intake in the high-protein groups was 1.81 grams per kilogram of body weight per day, more than double the recommended daily allowance according to most guidelines. The researchers found no evidence of harm. Increased protein intake did not negatively affect the *glomerular filtration rate,* a key marker of kidney function, nor was there any dose-response relationship indicating that higher protein levels caused damage.

Even in people with type 2 diabetes, a group more vulnerable to kidney issues, high-protein diets showed no adverse effects. Additionally, longer-term studies up to fifty-two weeks confirmed that higher protein consumption did not compromise kidney health. The findings challenge long-standing concerns about high-protein diets, suggesting that higher protein intake poses no significant risk to kidney function for healthy individuals.

Think of Protein as the Anchor Point in Your Diet

Unlike carbs and fats, protein needs are based on body weight, not energy expenditure. This means protein requirements are relatively stable from day to day. The evidence indicates that 1.2 to 1.4 grams of protein per kilogram of body weight (0.54 to 0.64 grams per pound) per day is a good target for general health.[328,333] If you're often hungry or focused on muscle growth, you could consider increasing it to 1.6 to 1.8 grams per kilogram (0.73 to 0.82 grams per pound).[328,333]

I'm generally not a fan of food tracking. However, providing you don't feel that monitoring your food intake could lead to or reinforce unhelpful eating patterns, some people find it useful to measure their protein intake for a couple of weeks to establish a baseline. Many apps are available that make it easy to record what you eat and automatically calculate the quantity of macronutrients. Once you've figured out how much protein you are eating on average, you can choose whether you want to adjust it.

* * *

Finally, besides protein *quantity*, it's important to consider *quality*. The recommendations I've shared assume that the protein consumed is high quality. A protein scoring system—the Digestible Indispensable Amino Acid Score (DIAAS)—provides some helpful guidelines to determine what high-quality means.[332] The score evaluates protein quality based on the availability of essential *amino acids*—the building blocks of protein that our body cannot produce on its own—and how effectively the body can absorb and use them. The higher the number, the greater the availability and digestibility.

FOOD	DIAAS
Whole milk	143
Milk protein concentrate	141
Whey protein concentrate	133
Ham (uncured)	124
Skim milk powder	123
Fish (flounder)	120
Beef jerky	120
Salami	120
Pork loin (medium-well done)	118
Bacon (smoked)	117
Pork loin (well done)	117
Egg (hard boiled)	113
Ribeye (roast, medium rare)	111
Fish (plaice)	110
Whey protein isolate	109
Chicken breast	108
Ribeye (well done)	107
Soy flour	105
Soy protein isolate	90
Chickpeas	83
Pea protein concentrate	82
Cooked rice	59
Tofu	52
Almonds	40
Rice protein concentrate	37

As you can see in the table, animal-based proteins tend to score highly, where plant-based proteins tend to score lower.[328,334] Animal proteins generally make it easier to consume sufficient high-quality protein, but this is also possible by eating a plant-based diet. Plant-based diets don't mean sacrificing adequate protein or performance, even among athletes. For example, a randomized controlled study compared recreational athletes' endurance and strength performance on three diets: plant based, plant based with meat alternatives, and omnivorous. After four weeks, no differences in running performance or muscle strength were observed across the groups, with all diets providing similar and sufficient protein intake.[335] It is important to note, though, that ensuring adequate, high-quality protein on a plant-based diet may require more intention, such as through variety, strategic food combinations, and possibly slightly higher total protein consumption.

To make the values that represent adequate, high-quality protein more tangible, imagine a 154-pound (70 kg) person aiming to consume 1.4 grams of high-quality protein per kilogram of body weight from both plant and animal sources—meaning they were aiming for about 100 grams of protein daily. This could look as follows:

Breakfast:

- 2 large eggs (13 g protein)
- 2 slices of whole grain toast (8 g protein)
- 1 cup milk (8 g protein)
- Total for breakfast: 29 g protein

Lunch:

- Grilled chicken breast (80 g) (24 g protein)
- ¾ cup cooked quinoa (6 g protein)
- Mixed greens with olive oil dressing (0 g protein)
- Total for lunch: 30 g protein

Snack:

- 1 medium apple with 2 tablespoons peanut butter (8 g protein)
- ½ cup almonds (14 g protein)

- 1 medium banana (1 g protein)
- Total for snack: 23 g protein

Dinner:

- Salmon fillet (100 g) (20 g protein)
- 1 cup steamed broccoli (3 g protein)
- 1 large sweet potato (4 g protein)
- Total for dinner: 27 g protein

Daily Total: 109 g protein

While spreading protein intake over the day in multiple meals can make hitting a target protein intake easier, it's not essential. It was once believed we needed to divide our protein intake into smaller amounts because of an upper limit to how much protein the body could absorb in a single sitting. However, more recent research has challenged this view. Very large protein doses, even up to 100 grams in a single sitting, may still be effectively utilized.[336] These findings suggest that we can divide our protein intake according to our routine or preferences. This could be based on one or two high-protein meals or smaller amounts of protein in more frequent meals and snacks.

There is no one-size-fits-all approach.

Fat Is Essential for Human Life

Carbohydrates have been called out as the enemy, and concerns about protein abound, but when it comes to unfair critiques of macronutrients, the discourse around fat is the archetype.

No one used to worry about fat until shortly after the Second World War, when new observational epidemiological research methods—which involve collecting data about what people are already doing—began to be developed. This led scientists to become more interested in population-level health.

Researchers noticed an association between saturated fat consumption and heart disease. Even though the research methods could only establish a correlation rather than causation, *biological plausibility bias* struck. The seemingly logical connection led many countries to launch population-level campaigns to reduce saturated fat intake. However, these campaigns didn't have the intended effect as rates of obesity and the incidence of cardiovascular disease continued to rise.

The link between fat and health is far more nuanced than early observational studies suggested. Newer research indicates that instead of fixating on total fat intake, we should focus on the types of fats we consume and the overall patterns of our diets.[337] As it turns out, fat isn't something to avoid—it's essential for human life.

Every cell in our body is encased in a phospholipid membrane—a flexible, double-layered barrier made of *fatty acids*. This membrane isn't just structural; it also plays a critical role in controlling what enters and exits each cell, protecting its contents and allowing essential nutrients to flow in while keeping harmful substances out.

Without sufficient dietary fat, our bodies struggle to build and maintain these vital cell membranes, affecting everything from brain function to immune health. Fats are also used to synthesize hormones, including estrogen, testosterone, and cortisol, and absorb some vitamins such as A, D, E, and K.

Industrial Food Processing Creates Most of the Problems

The potential for harm emerges when humans start messing around with the molecular structure of fats through industrial processing. For instance, *trans* fats—formed by a chemical process that turns liquid oils into solid fats—were introduced to improve the commercial performance of foods, increase shelf lives, and modify the fat structure to create specific textures and appearances.

While they are being phased out in some countries, trans fats are present in many ultraprocessed foods, such as partially hydrogenated oils in margarine, fast foods, and industrially produced baked goods. A 2 percent absolute increase in energy intake from trans fats has been associated with a 23 percent increase in cardiovascular risk.[338] It may be impossible for some people to avoid trans fats entirely, but we would benefit from limiting consumption of trans fats to a maximum of 2 grams per day.[338] To put this in context, a single donut could contain 1 to 2 grams of trans fat if it was made with partially hydrogenated oils.

Don't Fear Natural Fats

While highly processed fats should be avoided, we should not fear minimally processed natural fats from whole foods.

Food sources such as meat and dairy, which contain saturated fat, are also an excellent source of protein and essential nutrients, making them a valuable part of many diets. Nonetheless, it's likely beneficial to bias fat intake in favor of polyunsaturated fats (found in nuts, seeds, and oily fish), monounsaturated fats (abundant in olive oil, avocados, and almonds, for example), and omega-3 fats (rich in salmon, flaxseeds, and walnuts), all of which are associated with numerous health benefits. Essential fatty acids—omega-3 (alpha-linolenic acid) and omega-6 (linoleic acid)—are particularly important, as they contribute to the structure and function of cell membranes, but the body cannot synthesize them.

While both omega-3 and omega-6 fatty acids are essential, maintaining a proper balance between them is crucial.[339] Omega-3 fatty acids are well known for their anti-inflammatory properties and cardiovascular benefits. Omega-6 fats, found in foods such as nuts and seeds, are also essential, but some research suggests that omega-6 can be pro-inflammatory if consumed in excess relative to omega-3. To achieve a healthier balance, prioritize foods rich in omega-3s (such as fatty fish, flaxseeds, and walnuts) and choose omega-6 sources that are less processed and come from whole foods (such as nuts and seeds) rather than refined vegetable oils.

The World Health Organization and other guidelines recommend that fats comprise 20 to 35 percent of total calories.[337] The lower limit ensures sufficient energy, essential fatty acids, and absorption of fat-soluble vitamins. The upper limit in dietary guidelines is primarily aimed at avoiding excess calorie consumption, which can lead to weight gain—as I mentioned earlier in this chapter, fat is very energy dense.

Do Calories Really Count?

The notion that *calories don't count* has gained popularity recently, coinciding with a deeper understanding of the complexities involved in how our bodies process food. Factors such as food quality, hormonal regulation, and gut health significantly influence how we absorb and utilize calories. For instance, two people eating the same meal might metabolize and store those calories differently because of individual differences in gut health or metabolism. Additionally, it's now widely acknowledged that calorie counts on packaging and menus can be imprecise—sometimes by a wide margin. Nonetheless, the balance between calories consumed and calories burned remains a fundamental factor in weight management.

The *laws of thermodynamics*—which govern how energy is conserved and transferred—cannot be subverted. These laws dictate that energy cannot be created or destroyed, only converted from one form to another. When applied to nutrition, this means that if we consume more calories (energy) than our body uses, the excess is stored as fat, leading to weight gain. Conversely, consuming fewer calories than we expend forces the body to use stored energy, resulting in weight loss.

The key is to balance both perspectives: Calories do count, but they need to be viewed within the broader context of food quality, metabolic health, and individual differences.

But while calories matter, strict calorie counting isn't essential. For some, tracking every calorie can reinforce unhelpful eating patterns. Yet others find that a brief period of calorie tracking offers clarity, highlighting how their energy intake compares with expenditure and revealing where most of their calories come from—insights that can inform smarter eating choices.

For instance, you might keep protein intake steady but boost carbohydrate intake on high-activity days, given its role as an efficient fuel source. Conversely, if you were stuck in meetings all day—you could lower overall calorie intake, focusing on nutrient-dense vegetables and protein-rich foods that keep you satiated without overshooting your energy needs.

Is Fasting a Fad, and Does Meal Frequency Matter?

In addition to *what* we eat, people are becoming more interested in *how* often we eat. But there seems to be little consensus. On the one hand, you have people suggesting that eating smaller meals more frequently "keeps metabolism high." On the other hand, you find those recommending eating as few meals as possible.

Hyperoptimizers, in particular, often promote highly disciplined eating schedules with complex-sounding explanations featuring hypotheses centering on metabolism and insulin sensitivity, often accompanied by pictures of their abdominal muscles. But as we've explored in previous chapters, we need to be cautious about falling into the traps of *biological plausibility bias, precision bias,* and the *seductive allure of neuroscientific explanations*. So what's really going on?

Meal Frequency Does Not Boost Metabolism

Let's start by tackling the myth that higher meal frequency boosts metabolism. The incorrect argument suggests that eating more aids weight loss by creating a *thermic effect*—the slight increase in calorie burn that occurs when we eat. Proponents claim that every time we eat, our metabolism speeds up to digest and process the food, meaning more frequent meals would theoretically result in more calorie burn throughout the day, but it's another classic illustration of *biological plausibility bias* in action—it sounds logical, so people assume it is true.

While it's true that digestion temporarily increases energy expenditure, the total calories burned are proportional to the amount of food eaten, not the frequency. Eating six small meals of three hundred calories each or three larger meals of six hundred calories each will generally result in the same thermic effect if the total calorie intake is identical. Thus, meal frequency alone doesn't increase metabolic rate or lead to weight loss unless we're in a calorie deficit.

Comprehensive analyses of research findings support this view. A review of hundreds of studies found no meaningful link between meal frequency and weight loss, nor any significant difference in metabolic rate between eating more frequent, smaller meals and fewer, larger meals.[340] Studies using advanced methods to track energy intake and expenditure in highly controlled environments add further confirmation.

Fasting Only Influences Weight If We Eat Less

Intermittent fasting (IF) and *time-restricted eating* (TRE), which both feature alternating periods of eating and fasting, are getting a lot of attention, particularly among the hyperoptimizers who pervade social media.

Common IF and TRE methods include the following:

16/8, which involves fasting for sixteen hours and eating during an eight-hour window each day.

5:2: Adherents eat normally for five days a week and significantly reduce calorie intake on the other two days.

Alternate-day fasting, where people cycle between days of normal eating and days of fasting or eating very few calories.

Hyperoptimizers often argue that these approaches accelerate fat loss and improve body composition by "reducing insulin levels" independent of a calorie deficit. The rationale behind this claim is based on insulin's role in fat storage: When we eat, insulin levels rise to help cells absorb glucose for energy. During this process, fat breakdown slows as insulin promotes energy storage. The argument goes that fasting lowers insulin levels for extended periods, allowing the body to burn more stored fat. They will even quote studies reporting IF "reduces insulin plasma levels by 13.25 micro-international units"—a measure commonly used to quantify hormone concentrations in the blood.[341] According to their theory, the longer the body remains in a low-insulin fasted state, the more fat it will burn. Sounds convincing, but this is another example of *biological plausibility* and *precision bias.*

Their proposed mechanism sounds logical, and stating a very specific number lends credibility, but proponents of this theory completely overlook the fundamental importance of a calorie deficit for fat loss. While fasting lowers insulin and may shift the body to use stored energy, fat loss ultimately depends on consuming fewer calories than the body expends. Low insulin levels alone do not drive fat loss without being in a calorie deficit. The evidence is clear that IF and TRE result in weight loss for one simple reason: People end up eating fewer calories than they expend.[342,343]

I appreciate that weight loss is not the only aim of IF and TRE. One popular recommendation is to conduct exercise in the morning in a fasted state (i.e., before breakfast) based on the notion that this will burn more fat, along with other advantages. While some people may prefer to work out before eating, either for convenience or because they feel more comfortable, fasted training is not associated with fat burning or body composition benefits.[344] Rather, training in a fasted state can make exercise feel more effortful and impair performance, particularly during high-intensity efforts.[345]

Doesn't Fasting Improve Mental Clarity?

Hyperoptimization gurus love to talk about how their fasts improve their sense of focus and enhance cognitive performance, often accompanied by a few images of brain scans to leverage the *seductive allure of neuroscientific explanations.*

Calorie restriction and fasting seem to be associated with temporary positive changes in some aspects of cognition, such as *inhibition*, which may make us less distractable. However, other aspects, such as *cognitive flexibility*, are impaired—a critical capability in knowledge work.[346] These findings raise questions about the suitability of fasting as a productivity hack for complex, knowledge-intensive tasks.

Does Fasting Boost Longevity?

Another popular claim is that fasting boosts longevity, based on a combination of animal studies and the finding that when energy availability in our body is low, processes that prioritize cell repair and energy use are activated.[347] This includes slowing down the production of new cells and shifting attention toward repairing damaged ones.

While there may be benefits, there are potential downsides. Fasting can lead to muscle loss, particularly as we get older.[348,349,350] Overall, the weight of evidence concerning the importance of preserving muscle mass for both health span and longevity is stronger and more extensive than evidence concerning potential benefits from fasting and calorie restriction. It's also worth considering that, even if calorie restriction could extend life, quality of life could be significantly diminished if we lack the strength to pursue activities that give life meaning.

As I described in chapter 1, the decision about whether any intervention is suitable for you depends on whether there is a *positive expected value* based on the magnitude and probability of benefits and risks relative to costs in your context.

Avoid Dysregulating Your Appetite:
Eat with Your Body Clock

Chrononutrition—aligning our eating patterns with our circadian rhythm—is a mild form of TRE that we would all likely benefit from, as our internal body clocks, our metabolism, and even our gut microbiome are deeply intertwined.[351]

As I mentioned in chapter 4, light is the most powerful zeitgeber—a time cue—as it directly influences the suprachiasmatic nucleus (SCN)—the body's master clock in the brain. Food, specifically meal timing, acts as a much weaker cue to the peripheral circadian clocks in internal organs such as the liver.[352,353]

This alignment was passive for most of human history, as most activities, including eating, occurred while there was natural light. However, introducing artificial light and longer working days led to much more irregular and often later mealtimes, which affected how our body digests food and regulates appetite.

For instance, *social jetlag*, leading to irregular sleep and wake times, affects the gut microbiome's composition negatively, increasing the growth of less favorable strains of bacteria.[18] Eating later (10:00 p.m.) rather than earlier (6:00 p.m.) causes an 18 percent increase in blood sugar levels after eating, even when people sleep enough.[354] When we don't sleep enough, our appetite is dysregulated, making us feel hungrier.[355] On top of that, short sleep duration increases our preference for sweet-tasting treats.[356]

In contrast, eating patterns that align with circadian rhythms are linked to better weight control and overall metabolic health. Early time-restricted eating (eTRE)—eating earlier in the day—has shown particular promise. eTRE can improve glucose tolerance, insulin sensitivity, and blood pressure.[343,350] In practice, this could involve limiting eating to a twelve-hour window (between 6:00 a.m. and 6:00 p.m., for example), consuming most calories earlier in the day (such as by having a relatively larger lunch and smaller evening meal), and avoiding late-night meals. Perhaps there's truth in the adage that you should eat your breakfast, share your lunch, and give your dinner to your enemy.

Depending on their chronotype, some people may shift their twelve-hour eating window slightly earlier or later. Still, the evidence suggests that we would all likely benefit from eating relatively earlier and sleeping adequately at consistent times. Rather than forcing ourselves into more extreme hyperoptimized patterns of restricted eating, these simple actions represent the most effective ways to support our health and natural appetite regulation.

Should I Be Supplementing My Diet?

No chapter on nutrition would be complete without mentioning supplements.

At the time of writing, the global market for nutritional supplements is estimated to be worth nearly $400 billion, representing a broad range of products, including concentrated sources of vitamins, minerals, nutrients, or substances designed to add to the diet.[357]

Supplement manufacturers' claims could lead you to think that any pursuit of health and peak performance must include supplementation. However, this view is driven more by effective marketing than hard evidence.

For example, many products are focused on providing high doses of certain vitamins and minerals. People incorrectly assume that more must be better, but *ceiling effects* usually kick in—increasing the dose beyond a certain point does not increase the benefits. Healthy individuals likely do not gain from vitamin or mineral supplementation unless they have been diagnosed with nutrient deficiencies.[358]

However, it's important to acknowledge the potential for deficiencies. For instance, vegan diets can be associated with the risk of vitamin B12 deficiency, as this vitamin is found almost exclusively in animal-source foods.[359] Further, many people worldwide are deficient in vitamin D.[360] In these cases, if confirmed by testing, supplementation to correct the deficiencies could be beneficial.

Do Antioxidant Supplements Work?

In the absence of a deficiency, consuming unnecessarily high amounts of vitamins is, at best, a waste of money. At worst it could cause harm. Certain vitamins—especially the fat-soluble vitamins A, D, E, and K—can be toxic in high doses.[361] You can have too much of a good thing. This is also true of antioxidant supplements, including vitamin E, which have shown no consistent benefit and can be harmful when used indiscriminately.[362] Antioxidant supplement blends, such as combinations vitamin E, C, and beta-carotene, may even blunt the effectiveness of some medications.[363]

Can Magnesium Supplementation Improve Sleep?

Concerning minerals, magnesium has gained popularity as a supplement for improving sleep and seems effective for improving sleep in older adults.[364] As people age, their gastrointestinal systems can become less efficient at absorbing magnesium from food, so this benefit is likely a function of the supplement addressing a deficiency. Supplemental magnesium is unlikely to offer a benefit beyond the placebo effect in the absence of a deficiency.

Some people may point to a recent randomized controlled trial that reported magnesium supplementation improved sleep quality.[365] However, the researchers did not measure the participants' magnesium status, so the benefits may have resulted from addressing underlying deficiencies. Also, it's worth noting that the research was funded by the supplement manufacturer used in the trial.

What About Biotics?

The role of *biotics*—various substances that support a healthy gut microbiome—is gaining traction as research highlights links to immunity, metabolic health, and overall well-being.[366] A whole food approach can provide many of these benefits naturally, leveraging dietary sources of *probiotics, prebiotics, synbiotics,* and *paraprobiotics.*

Probiotics: Live Microbial Allies

Probiotics—live bacteria beneficial to gut health—are traditionally sourced from fermented foods. Yogurt, kefir, sauerkraut, and kimchi provide strains such as *lactobacillus* and *Bifidobacterium,* which can bolster digestion and immune function. A whole food diet rich in these fermented items introduces diverse microbes that may enhance gut resilience.

Prebiotics: Nourishing the Microbiome

Prebiotics are indigestible fibers that feed beneficial bacteria, as described earlier in the chapter, promoting a balanced microbiome. Foods high in prebiotic fibers, such as garlic, onions, leeks, bananas, and oats, stimulate bacterial growth and activity. Including these foods in meals nourishes gut microbes, fostering a healthy bacterial environment.

Synbiotics: Combining Forces

Synbiotics combine probiotics and prebiotics in a single product, designed to maximize the survival and activity of beneficial bacteria. While synbiotic supplements offer convenience, achieving similar effects through diet is possible. For instance, pairing yogurt (probiotics) with fiber-rich fruits such as bananas (prebiotics) may create a natural food-based synbiotic effect.

Paraprobiotics: Nonliving, Active Benefits

Paraprobiotics are inactivated microbial cells that may still exert health effects by modulating immune responses and reducing inflammation. Found in some pasteurized or heat-treated fermented foods, paraprobiotics can offer a gentler alternative for those sensitive to live probiotics.

Some research indicates that biotic supplementation may help maintain a healthy balance of gut microbes, which is linked to improved immune function and protection against various lifestyle-related diseases.[366] Yet while studies on animals and humans show promising connections, there is still no consensus on the ideal dosage needed to maximize benefits.

The bottom line is that healthy people without deficiencies, who eat varied, nonrestrictive diets featuring adequate energy and sufficient protein and are rich in fresh, minimally processed foods, are unlikely to benefit from routine vitamin, mineral, or biotic supplementation.[358] As always, though, there are exceptions. One such example is *creatine*.

Creatine: A Supplement That May Be Worth Considering

Creatine is a naturally occurring compound, primarily found in muscle cells, that plays a key role in producing energy during short bursts of high-intensity activity. The body can synthesize creatine in the liver and, to a lesser extent, the kidneys and pancreas. Creatine is also present in foods such as red meat and fish. However, supplementation can boost muscle creatine stores beyond what diet alone typically provides.

Creatine has become one of the most well-researched supplements, featuring in over five hundred peer-reviewed publications, demonstrating significant benefits for several aspects of health and performance.[367]

For Athletes and Fitness Enthusiasts

Creatine can enhance physical performance in sprinting and resistance exercise.[368] Research indicates that creatine supplementation, combined with resistance training, significantly enhances muscle strength.[369]

For Vegetarians and Vegans

Creatine is primarily found in animal products such as meat and fish, so vegans and vegetarians often have lower muscle creatine levels. In this case research suggests that creatine supplementation can be particularly beneficial, supporting cardiovascular health and athletic performance.[370,371]

For Older Adults

In older adults creatine has shown potential in combating age-related muscle loss and improving bone health. Some studies even indicate potential cognitive benefits.[367]

As for safety, creatine is one of the most extensively researched supplements, including in long-term, multiyear studies. It has shown no evidence of causing kidney, liver, or heart damage in healthy individuals, nor does it lead to dehydration or muscle cramps, as some myths suggest.[367] While it's possible to source creatine in whole foods, its concentration is much lower than in supplements. For example, you would need to eat a kilogram of beef to get the 5 gram dose, which is typical in many creatine supplementation protocols.[367]

With that said, I still recommend consulting a qualified health-care provider to seek advice before beginning supplementation, particularly for those with underlying health conditions or who are taking any medications.

When It Comes to Supplementation, Test, Don't Guess

Despite the potential benefits of some supplements, I urge people to be cautious. Unlike pharmaceuticals, most supplements are not rigorously tested for safety and efficacy before they reach the market. I'm not denying that people have positive experiences, but the evidence indicates that, with few exceptions, this is likely due to the correction of a deficiency or the placebo effect. If you think you may benefit from supplements, test, don't guess—speak to an appropriately qualified medical professional and explore whether assessment for deficiencies is an appropriate option.

How Much Do Dietary Needs Vary?

As we begin to wrap up this chapter, the following important unanswered questions remain:

1. How much do dietary needs vary from person to person?
2. How do you determine what works best for you?

A recent study featuring 2,000 participants revealed that each person has repeatable and predictable nutritional responses to different foods and that these differences vary between people, even between identical twins.[372] One of the largest randomized controlled trials on personalized nutrition conducted across seven European countries with over 1,600 adults also found that tailored dietary advice led to more substantial improvements in healthy eating behaviors than general guidelines.[373,374]

Participants who received personalized advice seemed to be better at sticking to their diets, which indicates that customization can support behavior change.[373,374] However, using more sophisticated—and often expensive—methods, such as genetic testing or body-type analysis to personalize the diets, did not seem to offer any specific benefits. The benefits are likely related to the increased human attention and support people receive in more sophisticated programs rather than any inherent superiority of the testing or technology.[375]

In other words, while research suggests no single, perfect, universally applicable diet exists, it is unlikely that advanced tools are necessary to identify what works to create a personalized eating plan.[373,374]

The best diet is usually the one you can stick to.

Until more definitive evidence emerges, it may be better to focus on looking for appropriately qualified people who can support you as you explore what approach to eating works best rather than seeking out sophisticated, costly, personalized nutrition strategies.

Be Your Own Scientist

We can take simple actions to personalize our diet without overcomplicating the process. One of the most straightforward is to conduct a series of personal experiments, beginning with the following three steps:

Start with One Change

Rather than overhauling your entire diet, try to pick one change that you can implement while keeping most other aspects of your life and work constant. For example, if your current diet includes a lot of processed food, begin by replacing these items with less processed, whole food options. Focus on this shift before considering more drastic changes such as eliminating entire food groups. Keeping most aspects of your lifestyle constant will help you isolate the effects of this one modification.

Define a Timescale

Changing dietary habits is notoriously challenging. By setting a clear, specific timescale—whether it's two weeks or two months—you create a structure that makes new habits easier to adopt. Knowing there's an end point can make even the toughest changes feel more manageable and less overwhelming.

Try to Measure the Effects

To track progress, decide how you'll measure the impact of your dietary changes. This could be as simple as keeping a journal of how you feel—monitoring your energy levels, mood, and stress. While we often rely on objective measures such as calories or nutrient intake, subjective well-being is one of the most reliable predictors of long-term health. Don't underestimate the power of feeling good.[376]

Fundamentally, humans are omnivores, capable of thriving on a wide variety of diets. This flexibility is part of what has allowed our species to flourish across different climates and ecosystems. While more research is needed to unlock the full potential of personalized nutrition, there's no need to get bogged down in the pursuit of the perfect diet.

An ongoing challenge is that some people are incentivized to make nutrition seem more complicated than it is. If they can get you to believe that the route to optimal health and performance is found in making precise adjustments to micro and macronutrients and supplement stacks, they can make themselves indispensable and sell you a whole range of products and services.

In reality, 99 percent of the benefits are found in ensuring that most of your meals come from minimally processed, natural, whole foods, eaten during the day (rather than late at night), combined with regular exercise and adequate, consistent sleep.

Now that doesn't mean you have to banish potato chips, chocolate bars, or soft drinks from your life. You can enjoy these things occasionally and still live a long, healthy, high-performing life. It's also worth reflecting on the fact that while these foods might not add much to your physical health, they can contribute to your social or psychological health. And that's a form of well-being worth considering, too.

Michael Pollan coined one of my favorite dietary guidelines back in 2007:

Eat food. Not too much. Mostly plants.[377]

In the end the goal isn't to chase perfection. It's to find a way of eating that supports your health and lifestyle while remaining adaptable and sustainable in the long run.

CHAPTER 6 REVIEW

In this chapter we explored why nutrition advice seems contradictory and ever changing. We examined how the challenging nature of nutrition research can lead to confusion when we try to apply findings, the effects of food processing, and how our circadian rhythms influence eating patterns. Rather than promoting a single perfect diet, we discovered evidence-based principles for making informed nutritional choices.

KEY INSIGHTS

FOOD PROCESSING LEVELS (NOVA CLASSIFICATION)

- **Unprocessed/minimally processed foods:** Natural foods with simple nonchemical changes.
- **Processed culinary ingredients:** Extracted directly from foods.
- **Processed foods:** Combining processed ingredients with unprocessed foods.
- **Ultraprocessed foods:** Products made primarily from food extracts and additives.

PROTEIN FUNDAMENTALS

- Aim for 1.2 to 1.4 g per kg of body weight daily.
- Higher-quality proteins score better on the DIAAS scale.
- Protein is more satiating than other macronutrients.
- Spreading intake throughout the day isn't essential.

CHRONONUTRITION PRINCIPLES

- Food timing acts as a circadian rhythm cue.
- Consider limiting eating to a twelve-hour window.
- Earlier eating is associated with better metabolic health.
- Late eating (10:00 p.m. versus 6:00 p.m.) can increase blood sugar by 18 percent.

SUPPLEMENT CONSIDERATIONS

- Most supplements are unnecessary for healthy people, but there are exceptions.

- Creatine shows consistent benefits across research.
- Test for deficiencies before supplementing.
- Vitamin and mineral excess can be harmful.

PRACTICAL ACTIONS

1. ASSESS FOOD PROCESSING

- Evaluate current diet using NOVA classification.
- Identify ultraprocessed food consumption.
- Plan gradual shifts toward less processed options.
- Focus on whole food sources.

2. CALCULATE PROTEIN NEEDS

- Determine daily protein target based on body weight.
- Assess current protein intake.
- Identify high-quality protein sources.
- Adjust intake if needed.

3. ALIGN EATING WITH CIRCADIAN RHYTHM

- Track current eating window.
- Consider earlier meal timing.
- Aim for consistent mealtimes.
- Avoid late-night eating.

Remember This

The best diet is usually the one you can stick to. Focus on minimally processed foods, adequate protein, and eating patterns that align with your circadian rhythm rather than chasing perfect optimization.

Looking Ahead

In our next chapter, we'll explore how to develop a regenerative mindset that helps us thrive under pressure.

CHAPTER 7

REGENERATIVE MINDSET: LEARN TO THRIVE UNDER PRESSURE

Work has become easier on our bodies but harder on our minds.

Over the past few decades, the physical demands of most jobs have significantly decreased: Automation has replaced tasks that once required muscle, and few people spend all day on their feet. However, the strain on our minds has increased. Employees feel like they are working harder and faster than ever to meet rising demands and pressures; one in four show signs of burnout.[378,379,380,381,382]

Reactions to this mental load are polarized. On one side, 68 percent of employees are disengaged and doing the bare minimum to get by.[80] At its extreme, this response is labeled the *soft life* (similar to *quiet quitting*), where avoiding stress and minimizing demands becomes the goal. On the other side lies *hustle culture*: the *hyperoptimizer-adjacent* ethic that glorifies long hours, embraces relentless work, and celebrates the belief that sheer willpower alone will overcome any obstacle. For its followers, discomfort is either ignored or reframed as a badge of honor based on the belief that "what doesn't kill me makes me stronger."

It's easy to caricature these responses: the *soft life* is often dismissed as laziness, while *hustle culture* is ridiculed as naive and possibly masochistic. Yet if we're honest, most of us have flirted with both approaches—either to escape the relentless pressures of *always-on* work or to convince ourselves that we just need to work harder for a few more weeks.

Rather than criticizing these extremes, it's worth considering that both are often well-intentioned coping mechanisms. The *soft life* offers a retreat from overwhelm, while *hustle culture* provides a sense of control in the face of unrelenting pressure.

While neither strategy is sustainable long term, instead of dismissing them, I'd like us to adopt a shoshin mindset—staying open and curious about what we can learn. Whether we lean toward the ease of the *soft life*, the grind of *hustle culture*, or find ourselves somewhere in between, exploring how these responses develop can help us discover a *third way* to handle pressure without sacrificing our well-being or performance.

A Couple of Caveats for This Chapter

Before we proceed, a couple of important caveats.

First, nothing in this chapter should be taken as mental health advice. Health issues and past traumas can shape how individuals respond to stress, and these situations require guidance from a qualified professional. This chapter is about understanding the general principles of how we respond to stress and exploring ways to improve performance under pressure rather than offering diagnoses or treatments.

Second, the responsibility for managing workplace pressure cannot rest solely on employees. People can't *yoga their way* out of feeling overwhelmed or dissolve their stress in fruit smoothies.[382] Organizations and leaders must be accountable for creating work environments that allow employees to meet their responsibilities without sacrificing their well-being, which often requires structural and cultural changes.

That said, stress and pressure are inevitable, even in the best workplaces. While some factors are out of our control, we often have more influence over stress than we think. Performing under pressure isn't an innate ability—it's a skill anyone can learn.

We'll explore how to strengthen this ability by focusing on the following four key areas:

Beliefs: Our understanding of stress and our assumptions about its impact.

Perceptions: How we interpret stressful situations.

Response: The physiological effects of stress on the brain and body.

Behavior: The actions we take when faced with stress.

Biased Measurement and Media Influence Can Shape Our Views

Our beliefs about stress are shaped by many influences, but two factors—how stress is measured and how the media reports on it—have an especially powerful impact.

Surveys designed to assess stress often lean toward measuring adverse outcomes, reinforcing a predominantly negative view of stress.[383,384] Additionally, the media amplifies this bias, as headlines highlighting harmful effects tend to attract more attention than nuanced stories about benefits. For example, a headline might read "One in four workers worldwide shows signs of burnout" rather than reporting "75 percent of employees *do not* feel burned out."

As a result, we are frequently exposed to information that frames stress as inherently damaging. This repetition strengthens existing beliefs about stress, but this doesn't necessarily mean everyone responds similarly.[385] In fact, responses tend to be polarized.

Repeated Messages Can Polarize Beliefs About Stress

For those who already view stress as harmful, streams of alarming statistics and headlines activate *confirmation bias*, further entrenching their beliefs. Each new warning reinforces their commitment to avoid pressure, validating their choice to pursue a low-stress, *soft life*.

On the other hand, people steeped in *hustle culture* often experience the *backfire effect*. Rather than reevaluating their stance, the barrage of negative messaging can prompt them to double down on their opposing view. For example, bombarding a hustler with warnings about stress will make them even more likely to embrace the "what doesn't kill me makes me stronger" mentality.

Social media algorithms intensify both biases, quickly curating content that reinforces existing beliefs and evokes strong reactions. But regardless of whether someone aligns with the *soft life* or *hustle culture*, their beliefs about stress set off a cascade of responses, starting with how they perceive stress.

Our Beliefs Skew Our Perception of Challenges

We perceive stress in the following two phases:

1. **Primary Appraisal:** This is your brain's first reaction to a situation. It asks three questions: (a) *Is this situation a threat to me? (b) Is it harmful or challenging? (c) Is it irrelevant?*[386] For example, if you're asked to give a big presentation, you might think, *This is scary! (a threat), or This will be hard (a challenge), or I don't care (it's irrelevant)*.

2. **Secondary Appraisal:** Following this initial reaction, your brain asks, *Can I handle this?* You consider whether you have the tools, skills, or resources to meet the demands of the situation.[387] For instance, you may consider yourself well prepared and feel confident for the presentation. Alternatively, you might sense that you didn't rehearse sufficiently and feel anxious.

Our beliefs influence what happens in these appraisal phases.

Soft life beliefs—where all stress is viewed as harmful—distort the *primary appraisal* phase, leading to consistent overestimation of the demands and harms associated with everyday tasks. This exaggerated sense of threat then spills into the *secondary appraisal* phase, causing people to underestimate their coping ability and leading to underconfidence.[388]

Hustle culture introduces a different kind of appraisal error. Instead of overestimating demands, the belief that *what doesn't kill me makes me stronger* can lead to underestimating risk in the *primary appraisal phase*.[389] This mindset cascades into *secondary appraisal*, causing people to overestimate their coping abilities, fostering overconfidence.[390]

While the *soft life* and *hustle culture* reinforce contrasting beliefs, resulting in different types of perception and appraisal errors, both philosophies set off a maladaptive cascade that disrupts how the brain regulates the body's stress response.

How the Brain Interprets and Coordinates
Our Stress Response

Humans have an incredibly sophisticated stress response. Imagine it as a symphony performed by an orchestra composed of different instruments, each arranged in sections. I'll explain the role of each section, but we need to begin by introducing the prefrontal cortex—the frontal lobe of the brain, which is responsible for many complex cognitive, emotional, and behavioral functions. While every section in the orchestra plays a vital role, the prefrontal cortex is the conductor. It doesn't control every note, but it decides which sections should lead and which should quiet down, balancing emotions, controlling impulses, and helping you focus.

Act One: A Dynamic Duo—the Prefrontal Cortex
and the Amygdala

The first part of the orchestra's performance focuses on a back-and-forth between the prefrontal cortex and the amygdala. The amygdala plays a key role in processing emotions, especially fear and anxiety. Think of the amygdala as the kettledrums in the orchestra—it reacts quickly, adding emotional depth and urgency. Ideally, the kettledrums follow the conductor's cues, playing louder or softer as needed. In this way the prefrontal cortex helps modulate emotional responses, keeping fear and stress in check.

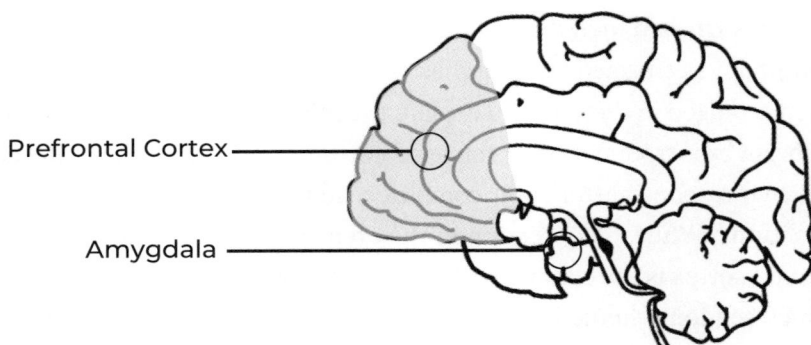

Prefrontal Cortex

Amygdala

However, faulty beliefs can disrupt this balance, leading to stress appraisal errors that amplify amygdala activity. Suppose we perceive all stress as a threat. Instead of drawing attention and adding emotion, the kettledrums perform on a hair trigger, leaping into action with an overwhelmingly high-volume, fast-tempo performance whenever there is a hint of tension.

When the amygdala becomes overactive—a phenomenon sometimes called an *amygdala hijack*—it can overpower the prefrontal cortex's ability to regulate the stress response, leading to a negative stress spiral.[391]

This is common in the *soft life* mindset, where overestimating demands and underestimating coping ability lead to an exaggerated stress response, followed by avoidance to try to stop it from happening in the future. I get it. No one wants to listen to kettledrums stealing the show.

In *hustle culture* the disruption works differently. Here, the prefrontal cortex may become overly focused on goal-directed behavior, allowing certain orchestra sections to dominate while neglecting signals from the amygdala.[392,393] The kettledrums play too fast and loud, but rather than sensing the performance is being disrupted, the high tempo might be perceived as motivating. However, over time, the relentless pace leads to chronic stress, altering brain function.[394]

Prolonged exposure to stress hormones can also disrupt the structure and function of the *hippocampus*, which connects emotions to memories.[395] As a result hustlers may have a harder time recognizing when their coping strategies are ineffective or noticing the early signs of excessive stress, perpetuating the cycle of overwork.

These misalignments in perception, prefrontal regulation, and amygdala activity set off a chain reaction that disrupts the activity of the next part of the performance, which focuses on the *hypothalamic-pituitary-adrenal (HPA) axis.*

Act Two: The (Dis)Harmony of the Hypothalamic-Pituitary-Adrenal (HPA) Axis

After the *prefrontal cortex* and the *amygdala* duet, the HPA axis comes into play.

Imagine the HPA axis as a critical three-instrument section in the orchestra composed of the *hypothalamus, pituitary gland,* and *adrenal glands.* Ideally, they complement one another perfectly. The *hypothalamus* is the first violin. It takes cues from the *amygdala* (its next-door neighbor in the brain orchestra), releasing *corticotropin-releasing hormone* to start the stress response.[396,397] The *pituitary gland* is the second violin. It responds to *corticotropin-releasing hormone* by secreting *adrenocorticotropic hormone.*[398] The *adrenal glands* are cymbals. Triggered by *adrenocorticotropic hormone,* they quickly discharge *cortisol* and *adrenaline,* increasing alertness, heart rate, and blood flow to prepare the body for action.[399,400]

The Hypothalamic-Pituitary-Adrenal (HPA) Axis

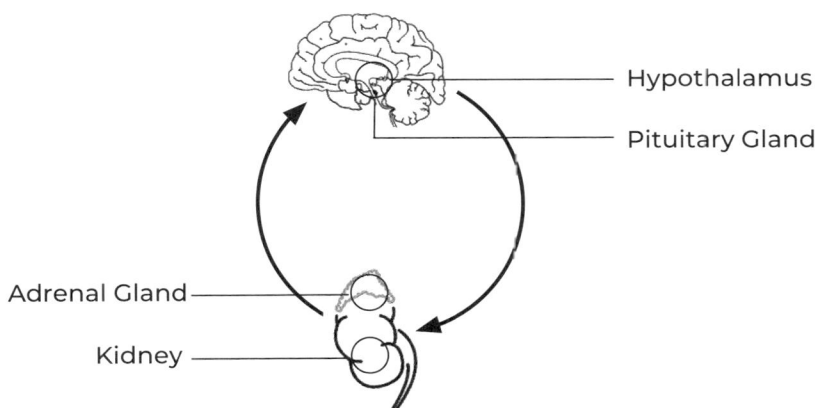

Hypothalamus
Pituitary Gland
Adrenal Gland
Kidney

The musicians in the HPA axis operate on a *negative feedback loop* to ensure they remain in harmony and the stress response does not continue indefinitely.[397,401] When we perceive a stress or challenge and the amygdala sounds the alarm, the HPA system ramps up to keep us alert and ready to handle challenges before gradually shutting down after the stressor diminishes or passes. However, this regulation mechanism can be disrupted by the *soft life* or *hustle culture*, albeit in different ways.

Act Three: The Soft Life and Hustle Culture Disrupt Our Stress Response

Some stress is necessary to maintain and fine-tune the HPA axis, like musicians who need to practice together.

However, consistently avoiding stress—as in an extreme pursuit of a *soft life*—can underactivate this system.[402] While this may feel desirable in the short term, repeated avoidance weakens stress resilience, leaving the brain and body less prepared to handle inevitable challenges.[403,404] Over time, this underuse of the HPA axis can result in exaggerated responses to minor stressors as the system loses its ability to modulate effectively.

In contrast, *hustle culture's* overconfidence traps people in a relentless cycle of stress, keeping the HPA axis constantly activated. This cortisol and adrenaline flood may feel productive, but it's like playing an orchestra at full volume without pause—eventually, the harmony collapses. We can observe this effect as chronic stress significantly worsens mental and physical health.[403,404]

Stress Can Bring Out Our Best and Worst Behavior

At the end of this chain reaction—beginning with our *beliefs,* shaping our *perceptions,* and activating our *physiological stress* response—we see how this cascade ultimately drives our *behavior.* Each step builds on the last, subtly yet powerfully, shaping how we react, make decisions, and act in response to stress.

Have you noticed that pressure can bring out the best or the worst in us?

Before we explore what can go wrong, take a moment to recall a time when you were truly at your best in a challenging situation—a time when stress energized you and brought out your natural talents. Think of a moment when you felt fully engaged, drawing on your strengths to meet the demands before you.

This could be at work, with friends, or during a personal project. Maybe you were solving a complex problem, showing kindness to someone in a difficult situation, or staying calm and self-regulated in the face of a challenge. These moments often reveal your *character strengths*—the positive qualities that come most naturally to you.

The character strengths framework incorporates twenty-four character strengths organized within six virtues.[405,406,407] We'll dive deeper into identifying and applying these strengths shortly. The key takeaway for now is that each of us has a unique profile of these strengths expressed across the six virtues. Think of this framework as a tool kit—each strength offers a practical way to navigate challenges.

VIRTUES	CHARACTER STRENGTHS
WISDOM	Creativity
	Curiosity
	Judgment
	Love of Learning
	Perspective
COURAGE	Bravery
	Perseverance
	Honesty
	Zest
HUMANITY	Love
	Kindness
	Social Intelligence
JUSTICE	Teamwork
	Fairness
	Leadership
TEMPERANCE	Forgiveness
	Humility
	Prudence
	Self-Regulation
TRANSCENDENCE	Appreciation of Beauty and Excellence
	Gratitude
	Hope
	Humor
	Spirituality

We Can Overuse and Underuse Our Character Strengths

In an ideal world, we would flawlessly harness our character strengths, finding the right balance every time. But of course, that's unrealistic—we're only human. The character strengths framework illustrates how we can all fall into patterns of *underusing* or *overusing* our strengths.[408] Picture a continuum, with the sweet spot for each strength in the center. At either end lie the dysfunctional extremes of underuse and overuse.

When stress and pressure mount, we're often pulled away from this balanced center, drifting toward these extremes. As a result strengths that would normally empower us can, in excess or neglect, hinder our well-being and performance.

Overuse And Underuse Of Character Strengths

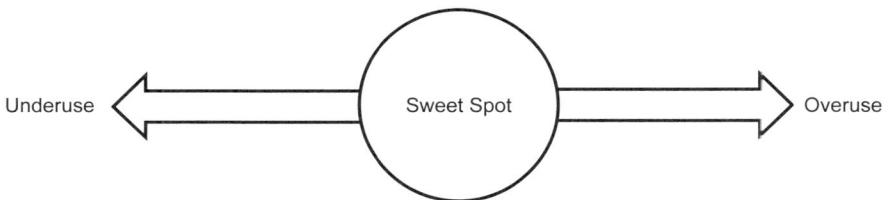

For example, in the *soft life*, overestimating threats, underestimating coping abilities, and exaggerated stress responses can lead to people spiraling into avoidance behaviors. This could look like an employee who views everyday responsibilities—such as giving a presentation or meeting a deadline—as overwhelming threats. Stress signals are perceived as fear rather than excitement or readiness to perform. Believing they can't handle the pressure, they disengage, avoid new challenges, and do the bare minimum to meet their job description, making it even harder to face difficulties in the future.

The character strengths framework describes this as an underuse of *courage* virtues such as *perseverance* or *bravery*. Over time, this underuse may create a sense of *learned helplessness*—reinforcing the belief that we have no control over stressful situations.[409]

Conversely, the belief that stress can be ignored in *hustle culture* fosters overconfidence, causing people to miss important stress signals and spiral into overwork and underrecovery. This could look like someone who takes on an ever-increasing number of projects, pushing themselves to meet tight deadlines and exceed expectations, framing every new task as a challenge to be conquered. However, they become overly confident handling mounting workloads, ignoring signs of fatigue or stress, believing that sheer effort will keep them ahead. The constant flood of stress hormones might even be misinterpreted as a necessary fuel for productivity, further reinforcing the cycle.

The character strengths framework describes this as overusing strengths such as *bravery* and *perseverance*, keeping the body's stress response in constant overdrive, potentially resulting in burnout.

These are just brief examples. Any character strength can be overused or underused, but to break free from these negative spirals, we need strategies that help us change beliefs, shift our perceptions, rebalance our stress response, and find the sweet spot for our character strengths.

Change Your Beliefs: Your Stress Mindset Can Shift in Minutes

Picture this: You're about to give a crucial presentation. Your heart races, your palms sweat, and your mind floods with worst-case scenarios. Conventional wisdom might suggest you should try to relax or ignore the feelings of stress. Not many people seem to believe that stress could be helpful.

When asked about the best advice for performing in stressful situations, 91 percent said staying calm was the best option.[410] But what if that advice is not just wrong but counterproductive? More than ten years of research have revealed that shifting our *stress mindset* by cultivating a broader belief that stress can have positive effects is a more successful and beneficial approach.[384,411] And it doesn't take too long or even require a huge amount of effort.

Alia Crum, a highly regarded Stanford University stress researcher, led a three-part study revealing how quickly our beliefs about stress can shift and how this can influence our health and performance.[411] To begin, the researchers validated a tool that could distinguish between two stress mindsets: *stress is enhancing,* characterized by people who believe that stress positively affects their performance, and *stress is debilitating,* where people believe stress has a negative impact.

Next, the researchers tried to change the participants' stress mindset, either positively or negatively, by sending three short (three-minute) educational videos via email over one week. The videos described the effects of stress in three different domains: health, performance, and personal development. One group received videos explaining the enhancing effects of stress in these domains, another received videos suggesting stress is debilitating, while a third group acted as a control.

In the final part of the study, the participants completed a public speaking exercise to examine how they performed under pressure.

The study confirmed that it's possible to measure whether someone holds a stress-is-enhancing or stress-is-debilitating mindset with a simple eight-question survey.

Assess Your Stress Mindset

If you're interested, you can try the survey for yourself. For each statement, rate the extent to which you agree or disagree on a scale from 0 to 4.

	STRONGLY DISAGREE	DISAGREE	NEITHER AGREE NOR DISAGREE	AGREE	STRONGLY AGREE
THE EFFECTS OF STRESS ARE NEGATIVE AND SHOULD BE AVOIDED.	4	3	2	1	0
	STRONGLY DISAGREE	DISAGREE	NEITHER AGREE NOR DISAGREE	AGREE	STRONGLY AGREE
EXPERIENCING STRESS FACILITATES MY LEARNING AND GROWTH.	0	1	2	3	4
	STRONGLY DISAGREE	DISAGREE	NEITHER AGREE NOR DISAGREE	AGREE	STRONGLY AGREE
EXPERIENCING STRESS DEPLETES MY HEALTH AND VITALITY.	4	3	2	1	0

	STRONGLY DISAGREE	DISAGREE	NEITHER AGREE NOR DISAGREE	AGREE	STRONGLY AGREE
EXPERIENCING STRESS ENHANCES MY PERFORMANCE AND PRODUCTIVITY.	0	1	2	3	4
	STRONGLY DISAGREE	DISAGREE	NEITHER AGREE NOR DISAGREE	AGREE	STRONGLY AGREE
EXPERIENCING STRESS INHIBITS MY LEARNING AND GROWTH.	4	3	2	1	0
	STRONGLY DISAGREE	DISAGREE	NEITHER AGREE NOR DISAGREE	AGREE	STRONGLY AGREE
EXPERIENCING STRESS IMPROVES MY HEALTH AND VITALITY.	0	1	2	3	4
	STRONGLY DISAGREE	DISAGREE	NEITHER AGREE NOR DISAGREE	AGREE	STRONGLY AGREE
EXPERIENCING STRESS DEBILITATES MY PERFORMANCE AND PRODUCTIVITY.	4	3	2	1	0
	STRONGLY DISAGREE	DISAGREE	NEITHER AGREE NOR DISAGREE	AGREE	STRONGLY AGREE
THE EFFECTS OF STRESS ARE POSITIVE AND SHOULD BE UTILIZED.	0	1	2	3	4

You may note that some questions are phrased negatively. However, I've already applied reverse scoring to these items, so use the values directly from the table to calculate your score as follows:

Average Your Ratings: Add up the ratings for all eight statements, then divide by eight to get your average.

Interpretation: Higher scores reflect a greater tendency toward a stress-is-enhancing mindset.

* * *

In addition to confirming that they could measure participants' stress mindset, the researchers discovered that simply watching the three short videos was sufficient to measurably shift the participants' beliefs about stress. The results also revealed that believing stress is enhancing was associated with participants seeking more detailed feedback, which could improve future performance, and more moderate cortisol reactivity, suggesting better regulation of the HPA axis.[411]

The stress-is-enhancing mindset intervention seemed to benefit a wide range of people—those who performed at their best with more stress and those who benefited from a smaller stress response.[411] This finding suggests this belief-shifting approach may be suitable, whether we tend toward *hustle culture*, the *soft life*, or somewhere in between.

Related research adds further support to these findings. For example, public speakers who adopt a stress-is-enhancing mindset and reappraise stress as exciting are rated more persuasive, confident, and competent by audience members.[410]

In an educational context, students who learned to reappraise stress before taking the GRE (a standardized test for graduate school admission) outperformed their peers on practice tests and the official exam months later.[412] Further, people with a stress-is-enhancing mindset report higher life satisfaction, lower anxiety and depression, and healthier physiological responses to stressors.[384]

Shifting Our Stress Mindset Has Long-Lasting Benefits

In a more recent study, Alia Crum and her team at Stanford set out to replicate the earlier findings and extend them.[383] As in the original research, the study attempted to shift the participants' beliefs rather than trying to eliminate or encourage people to endure stress. However, this time the researchers tested a novel approach called a metacognitive intervention—essentially, teaching individuals to think about how they think about stress.

The intervention was designed to help people shift to a more positive mindset, even in the face of conflicting information, such as the media messages suggesting that all stress is bad for you. As in the earlier study, the intervention changed how people viewed stress, improving health markers and work performance. These benefits were observed across different work environments, and the intervention was effective whether it was delivered as live training or online via twelve short videos.

Perhaps most encouraging, the mindset shift was durable. Unlike traditional approaches that might briefly alter thinking, this method created lasting change, even when participants were later exposed to information reinforcing negative views of stress. The positive effects remained eight months later—even during the early stages of the COVID-19 pandemic, when stress levels and negative messages were at an all-time high.

Rethink Stress with These Simple Steps

If you're curious to try it, you can find Crum's *Rethink Stress* course, which was used to shift participants' stress mindset, on the Stanford University Mind and Body Lab website.[413]

The following steps could also help you rethink your beliefs and reappraise your stress response, turning it into a tool for growth rather than something to avoid or ignore:

> **Explore the paradox of stress:** Seek out information demonstrating that stress can have both enhancing and debilitating effects. This more nuanced view sets the stage for a mindset shift. For instance, if you believe all stress is harmful, read studies showing that stress boosts resilience and performance.[384,411,414] If you think stress is purely mental and can be ignored, consider research on the physical effects of chronic stress.[394,403,404]

> **Think about thinking:** Recognize that we all have a particular mindset about stress—a set of beliefs and ideas you hold to be

true—and that this mindset can be changed. This awareness is key to the process.

Learn about the impact of your stress mindset: Search for content that reveals how mindsets can powerfully influence our performance, health, and personal development, such as the studies referenced in this chapter and the *Rethink Stress* course.

Acknowledge stress: When facing a stressor (e.g., a big presentation), label the experience as stress rather than trying to suppress or ignore it. This conscious cognitive process can activate prefrontal brain regions associated with deliberate thought rather than reactive fight-or-flight responses.

Welcome stress: Instead of avoiding, ignoring, or trying to reduce stress, reinterpret your stress response as a signal that something you value is at stake. For instance, noticing that your heart rate is elevated and that you feel nervous before a big presentation signals that you care about your performance and the impact you will have on the audience.

Utilize stress: Develop strategies to harness stress as an energy source to tackle the demands causing the stress. For example, you could reappraise pre-event nervousness as excitement and enthusiasm, which you could use to elevate your performance and convey your passion for the topic.

Create implementation intentions: Plan specific cues (e.g., feeling your heart rate increase) that will trigger your new stress response (e.g., "This energy will help me perform better"). This can enhance your sense of competence and trust in your coping ability.

Practice regularly: Use daily anchors to practice your new approach to stress. For example, each time you step out your front door, visualize the process of reframing the sensations of stress as fuel for your performance. This repetition builds and strengthens the neural pathways for your new response. High-quality research reveals that frequently using cognitive reappraisal has a durable, causal effect on improving mental health outcomes and reducing negative perceptions of stress.[415]

Reflect and review: Periodically assess how your new mindset affects your performance, health, and well-being. Use these insights to refine your approach.

Maintain perspective: Remember that adopting a stress-is-enhancing mindset doesn't mean seeking out unnecessary stress but rather enhancing your response to inevitable challenges.

Beware of Echo Chambers Reinforcing Unhelpful Beliefs

We must also recognize the risk of echo chambers—environments that reinforce our beliefs while subtly discouraging us from exploring other perspectives. As the introduction to this chapter notes, social media algorithms amplify this effect by feeding us content aligned with our existing interests and predispositions, narrowing our exposure to alternative viewpoints.

Breaking out of these echo chambers can be both eye-opening and beneficial. If you view stress as harmful and are drawn to a *soft life* approach, consider having a conversation with a friend or colleague who thrives in high-pressure situations. Alternatively, if you lean toward *hustle culture,* seek insights from those who prioritize rest; their perspective may reveal strategies to manage stress more sustainably.

Embracing this open-minded, nondual thinking helps counter *confirmation bias* and reduce the *backfire effect,* fostering a more adaptable perspective on stress. This approach isn't about denying the potential adverse effects of chronic stress. Instead, it's about learning to engage with stress in a healthier way, recognizing it as a part of life to be navigated—not something to be entirely avoided or ignored.

Try Some Evidence-Based Stress Management Techniques

In addition to shifting our mindset and reappraising stress, several complementary approaches can positively influence how our brain and body coordinate our stress response. There is an almost endless range of interventions to choose from, so we will look at four supported by good evidence, which are relatively simple to integrate into every day: *sleep, exercise, mindfulness meditation, and breathing exercises.*

1. GET SOME OVERNIGHT THERAPY

In chapter 4, I highlighted the bidirectional relationship between sleep and stress: Stress can interfere with sleep, and not sleeping enough can elevate stress.[159] Shortening sleep heightens activity in the amygdala, amplifying our stress responses.[207,214] In contrast, adequate sleep helps regulate amygdala activity. This supports the stress appraisal process, making it more likely that we'll perceive challenges as positive, or something we can cope with, rather than overwhelming.[416]

While we don't always make the connection, sleeping enough at a relatively consistent time is the foundation for a healthy, adaptive stress response. As I mentioned in chapter 4, sleep is so critical for regulating emotions that it has been characterized as *overnight therapy.*[207] As a starting point, I encourage you to apply the sleep tips I shared in the sleep chapter, but don't hesitate to seek support from an appropriately qualified professional if you struggle with sleep. There are many effective interventions available.

2. STRESS-PROOF YOURSELF WITH EXERCISE

In chapter 5 I described the benefits of physical activity and exercise for mental health, such as how simply taking a twenty-one-minute walk each day could lower the risk of depression by 18 percent[263] and how regularly exercising for 150 minutes per week at moderate intensity—equivalent to a brisk walk for most people—had the same impact on depression as taking an antidepressant.[276]

Exercise positively affects several brain structures that help regulate emotions and behavior. For example, regular exercise can bias activity in the amygdala toward feelings of happiness and against fear.[417] Just thirty minutes of aerobic activity, like brisk walking or jogging at 60 to 70 percent of your maximum heart rate, can increase activity in the *hippocampus,* a region crucial for memory and emotion regulation.[54]

Exercise also has an acute stress-buffering effect. People who exercised before facing a stressful task reported feeling better and recorded lower levels of *cortisol,* the body's primary stress hormone.[54] Together, these various forms of evidence point to exercise having a *stress inoculation effect,* where regular exercise can improve our ability to handle both physical and psychological stress.[418,419,420]

3. CONSIDER MINDFULNESS

Mindfulness has gone mainstream and is increasingly promoted as a solution for coping with our high-stress, always-on world. But despite its popularity, there is still no universally accepted definition of *mindfulness meditation* or agreement about precisely what mindfulness involves.[421] For this chapter we'll define *mindfulness meditation* as the practice of paying attention to the present moment without judgment.

The lack of a single definition has not curtailed the growth of mindfulness research, and many findings are positive. A review of forty-seven trials featuring over three thousand participants found that mindfulness interventions are moderately effective in reducing symptoms of anxiety and depression.[422] An analysis of thirteen studies featuring over two thousand participants observed that, when compared with people who took no action, participating in group-based, teacher-led mindfulness sessions was generally associated with decreased psychological distress.[423]

Several studies have also revealed that mindfulness meditation can change our brain structure, particularly in relation to gray matter, which makes up about 40 percent of brain tissue.[424,425] Some of the most consistent neuroscientific evidence indicates that meditation practice affects the right anterior ventral insula—a small, deep part of the brain near your ear. This structure plays a crucial role in processing emotions and feelings, suggesting that meditation may particularly affect areas involved in emotional regulation.[424] However, despite these positive findings, the evidence is not quite as strong and unequivocal as it is sometimes presented.

Mindfulness Under the Microscope: How Strong Is the Evidence?

One critical issue is that most mindfulness studies feature small sample sizes.[421,424,426] This characteristic makes it unclear whether a general population will experience benefits like those who participated in the study.

Also, most mindfulness research features cross-sectional study designs.[421,424,426] This means researchers only observe participants at a single point in time, capturing a snapshot of their mindfulness practices and outcomes. While this approach can identify associations—like a link between mindfulness and lower stress—it cannot prove causation. In other words, we can't be sure if mindfulness is directly causing the observed effects or if other factors may influence the results.

Are Mindfulness Brain Changes Meaningful or Just Seductive Science?

Media outlets and influencers are particularly fond of reporting on changes in brain structures associated with meditation practice. However, whether these changes are directly associated with meaningful effects in the real world is still unclear. There is a risk that we may fall victim to *biological plausibility bias*—assuming a logical explanation proves causation—and the *seductive allure of neuroscientific explanations*—the observation that we find explanations more convincing and satisfying simply because they contain neuroscientific terms.[49]

Is Mindfulness the Most Appropriate Tool?

Another key challenge is that only 9 percent of mindfulness research has compared mindfulness with active controls.[421] This means that most studies compared mindfulness practice with doing nothing. As a result, the effects may appear larger than they are in practice, where people may be able to choose another stress management technique rather than mindfulness being their only option. Further, the lack of active controls means it is impossible to determine if other interventions could be equally or perhaps more effective.[427]

For example, research suggests that fostering hope may be more effective than mindfulness in helping people cope with prolonged workplace stress, highlighting the value of looking ahead over simply staying in the moment when navigating challenging times.[428]

Finally, it's important to note that mindfulness is not entirely without potential risks. For example, in some people, mindfulness practices can increase anxiety and worsen some mental health outcomes.[429] However, less than 25 percent of mindfulness studies actively measure adverse effects, so we still don't have a clear idea about the downsides.[422,430]

I'm certainly not against mindfulness. Evidence and anecdotes indicate it is worth keeping in the stress management toolbox. For instance, mindfulness and *positive* reappraisal—the ability to reframe stressful events in a more positive light—appear to work in tandem, creating an upward spiral that reduces stress and enhances well-being.[431]

Nonetheless, while mindfulness can be effective, much remains to be learned. We need more randomized controlled trials and longitudinal studies with larger sample sizes to establish the benefits of mindfulness more definitively.[421,424,426] This research may also help us better understand which types of mindfulness work best for different people and identify when other approaches may be more effective.

4. USE BREATHING TO RECALIBRATE YOUR STRESS RESPONSE

Controlled breathing, where the pace and depth of inhalations and exhalations are consciously controlled, is an aspect of several mindfulness interventions. However, controlled breathing can be very effective in isolation.

In chapter 3 I mentioned how controlling our breathing can shift brain activity and adjust physiological responses to promote relaxation, improve mood, decrease blood pressure, and reduce cortisol levels.[176,177] I also introduced a simple breathing exercise and described how, when we breathe slowly and rhythmically, the expansion and contraction of our lung tissue increase vagus nerve activity.[179,180] This stimulation of the vagus nerve shifts the nervous system toward a parasympathetic *rest-and-digest* state, increases power in *alpha band* brain wave frequencies, and decreases *theta power*, which is associated with reduced tension and anxiety.[181,182,183]

Controlled breathing can be effective across a wide range of patterns and durations.[177] If you're curious to try controlled breathing, provided you don't have any health conditions that may prevent or make it risky, you could experiment with the breathing pattern that I introduced in chapter 3 as a starting point. Other breathing patterns, such as *symmetric pattern breathing*, also show promise for improving well-being and performance. For example, in one study, participants inhaled for a count of five, held their breath for a count of two, and then exhaled for a count of five, for just two minutes. This practice was associated with improved performance in a challenging decision-making task (nearly 50 percent more correct responses) and reduced perceived stress.[432] Overall, it seems that simple, controlled breathing techniques are one of the most reliable ways to positively influence how our nervous system responds to stress and performs under pressure.[177]

Which Stress Management Technique Is Most Effective?

Whenever I deliver a keynote or workshop on the topic of performing in high-pressure contexts, I'm often asked the same question: "Which stress management technique is most effective?"

My answer is always the same: It depends. However, some comparative research offers a helpful perspective. For example, a recent study observed that a daily five-minute breathwork session featuring deep inhalations, followed by slower, extended exhalations improved mood and reduced anxiety to a greater extent than mindfulness meditations of a similar duration.[433]

The study had some limitations. For example, the meditation sessions may have needed to be longer for benefits to emerge. However, if you are pressed for time, the study supports using brief breath control exercises to manage stress and mood during the day.

Another study compared three methods: twenty minutes of physical activity, a mindfulness meditation workshop, or heart rate variability biofeedback—a technique that involves breathing at a specific pace guided by technology, such as HRV4Biofeedback: a smartphone app that is available in most app stores.[434] All three interventions reduced perceived stress, decreased anxiety, and improved psychological well-being to a similar extent.

Personally, among these three techniques, I would generally favor exercise if you're short on time. My reasoning is that exercise likely represents the best return on investment because of its combined physical and psychological benefits. As little as twenty minutes of moderate-intensity exercise (65 to 70 percent VO_2 max) can reduce stress, decrease inflammation, and improve cognitive function.[54,435]

Ultimately, the choice is yours. The best stress management technique is the one that works best for you.

Perform at Your Best Under Pressure

Shifting your mindset, reappraising stress, and rebalancing your stress response, whether with sleep, exercise, mindfulness, or paced breathing, can all help you steer clear of the extremes of the *soft life* or *hustle culture*. These practices can also build resilience and support sustainable performance.

The final step—recalibrating our character strengths—ensures we can perform at our best when demands are high.

As we explored earlier, when we're under pressure, the positive qualities that come most naturally to us can be overused or underused, making them work against rather than for us. Underuse and overuse of our *character strengths* are associated with several adverse outcomes, such as lower life satisfaction and worse mental health.[408]

In contrast, the ideal use of character strengths correlates with improved well-being and performance under pressure.[408] For example, using strengths such as *creativity*, *curiosity*, and *love of learning* is strongly associated with positive coping strategies in the face of stress.[436] Emotional and interpersonal strengths such as *bravery, persistence, hope, kindness,* and *social intelligence* are linked to more active, problem-focused coping, such as seeking support and maintaining relationships rather than avoidance.[436] These strengths help people perceive stressful situations more clearly, develop new problem-solving approaches, and learn the appropriate lessons from challenges, fostering healthy confidence.

The balanced use of character strengths also has a stress-buffering effect, protecting us from some of the adverse effects of work pressure, particularly in high-stress occupations.[436] For instance, after experiencing a stressful situation, the heart rate and blood pressure values of people who can better express strengths related to *caring, inquisitiveness,* and *self-regulation* recovered more quickly.[437] Finding opportunities to use *signature strengths* (our top-ranked character strengths) in challenging situations can also improve people's ability to cope, boost mood, and enhance performance.[438,439,440]

The *sweet spot* in our character strengths—where we use them just the right amount—is sometimes described as the *golden mean.*[408]

The Golden Mean: How to Find the Sweet Spot for Your Character Strengths

Finding this *golden mean* may seem elusive, but good evidence indicates that we can develop and train our ability to use our character strengths in an ideal zone to increase our ability to perform under pressure.[405,408] The first step is to identify your top character strengths.

The VIA Institute on Character—a nonprofit organization dedicated to bringing the science of character strengths to the world—offers a free scientifically validated character strengths assessment on its website.[441] Once you've identified and familiarized yourself with your character strengths, research offers the following practical strategies to help you develop them and find your *golden mean*[408]:

> **Engage in strengths spotting:** Develop your *strengths fluency*—the ability to recognize, understand, and apply your and others' character strengths effectively—by paying more conscious attention

to how you and others use your character strengths in different situations. For example, a project manager could make a habit of noting how team members use their strengths during meetings or in their work outputs. They might notice how one team member consistently uses their strength of *creativity* to develop innovative solutions while another uses their strength of *social intelligence* to smooth over conflicts.

Seek feedback: Our self-perception of whether we have hit the *golden mean* for our character strengths can be biased. Caring, constructive, and honest input from others can provide a helpful perspective. For instance, a marketing analyst might think they're using their strength of *judgment* effectively, but colleagues might perceive it as overly negative criticism. We can better understand how our strengths are perceived and used in different contexts by actively seeking feedback, perhaps through regular check-ins or a 360-degree review process.

Practice mindfulness: Mindfulness may not be a cure all, but it seems effective in helping people notice when they are overusing or underusing their character strengths. This could involve taking brief pauses throughout the day to check in with yourself. For example, a software developer might realize they've been hyper-focused on solving a coding problem for hours without a break, potentially overusing their strength of *perseverance*, resulting in excessive sedentary time. Mindfulness could help them recognize this and take a step back to reassess their approach or take a movement break.

Use the tempering effect: Deliberately engage a balancing strength when you notice you're overusing a strength. For example, use *self-regulation* to temper overused *curiosity*. A researcher with a strong *curiosity* strength might find themselves constantly starting new projects without finishing old ones. They could consciously use *self-regulation* strength to set boundaries and focus on completing tasks before moving on to new interests.

Try the towing effect: Use your top strengths to bolster underused ones. Imagine a data scientist with a strong *love of learning* who wants to develop more *gratitude*. They could use their love of learning to research the benefits of gratitude and try proven interventions to improve it, such as gratitude lists.[442]

Put These Ideas into Practice

These ideas for developing and using character strengths can be summed up in the *AEA model*.

Aware: Build awareness by identifying key strengths through the VIA Survey, using the results to create a common language around these strengths.

Explore: Reflect on how your strengths have shaped past and current experiences, gaining deeper insight into how your strengths influence your actions, energy, and responses to challenges.

Apply: Create an action plan to actively use your character strengths in daily life, building on themes from the exploration phase and applying them in concrete, practical ways.

Repetition of these steps helps reinforce and build momentum in character strength development.

Finding our *golden mean* with character strengths requires ongoing reflection and fine-tuning. However, by cultivating awareness and practicing the application of our strengths across different contexts, we can harness their potential and improve our ability to perform under pressure.

Conducting the Symphony of Performance Under Pressure

Our ability to perform under pressure is a complex symphony.

I encourage you to recognize that you can change your beliefs and stress mindset, regardless of what the audience—the people looking on and the media—are saying. Acknowledge that our *primary* and *secondary stress appraisals* are simply the opening movements, setting the tone but not determining the entire composition. Try to make time to do the things that will help the orchestra—your brain and body—respond flexibly and healthily to stress.

If the music is in time and tune, you'll find it much easier to allow your signature strengths to shine in solo moments but also learn when to let them rest.

By adopting a shoshin beginner's mind, we can become open and ready to adapt to the nuances of each performance. The goal is not to avoid stress entirely or to constantly push through it but to create a masterful composition that resonates with your true potential. By embracing the full spectrum of your capabilities, you can tackle whatever challenges come your way.

CHAPTER 7 REVIEW

In this chapter we explored how work has become easier on our bodies but harder on our minds, with one in four showing signs of burnout. We examined how reactions to this mental load have become polarized—between the *soft life* that avoids all stress and *hustle culture* that glorifies relentless work. Through understanding how our beliefs about stress, our perceptions, and our physiological responses interact, we discovered evidence-based approaches to perform better under pressure while protecting our well-being.

KEY INSIGHTS

THE STRESS RESPONSE SYSTEM

- The prefrontal cortex acts as the conductor.
- Our amygdala processes emotions and fear.
- The HPA axis coordinates our physiological response.
- These systems work together like an orchestra.

STRESS APPRAISAL PROCESS

- **Primary Appraisal:** Is this threatening, challenging, or irrelevant?
- **Secondary Appraisal:** Can I handle this?
- Our beliefs influence both appraisal phases.
- Appraisal errors can lead to maladaptive responses.

CHARACTER STRENGTHS FRAMEWORK

- Twenty-four character strengths are organized into six virtues.
- Strengths can be overused or underused.
- Finding the sweet spot is key.
- Balance is needed between different strengths.

EVIDENCE-BASED STRESS MANAGEMENT

- Sleep regulates amygdala activity.
- Exercise has a stress-buffering effect.
- Mindfulness shows moderate effectiveness.
- Controlled breathing can shift nervous system state.

PRACTICAL ACTIONS

1. CHANGE YOUR STRESS MINDSET

- Notice and label stress responses.
- Reframe stress as *performance energy*.
- Create implementation intentions to anticipate your response.
- Practice reappraisals in everyday life.

2. FIND YOUR CHARACTER STRENGTHS BALANCE

- Identify signature strengths.
- Watch for overuse and underuse.
- Use the *tempering effect*—balancing out strengths—when needed.
- Apply the *towing effect*—use stronger strengths to support weaker ones.

3. BUILD YOUR STRESS MANAGEMENT TOOL KIT

- Prioritize adequate sleep.
- Include regular exercise.
- Consider mindfulness practice.
- Use controlled breathing techniques.

Remember This

Stress isn't inherently good or bad—it's how we perceive and respond to it that matters. Finding the sweet spot in our character strengths helps us perform better under pressure.

Looking Ahead

In our final chapter, we'll explore how to undo the distortions of *hustle culture* and the *soft life* to create sustainable growth.

CHAPTER 8

REGENERATIVE GROWTH: UNDOING THE DISTORTIONS OF HUSTLE CULTURE AND THE SOFT LIFE

Despite the relentless growth of the self-improvement industry, we're less satisfied than ever.

In this final chapter, the rubber hits the road—we're diving into how to turn good intentions into growth and lasting change. But before we get there, it's crucial to understand why so many self-help methods fall short.

The self-improvement market is booming, encompassing everything from personal development and wellness to career, relationship, and spirituality advice.[443] The industry thrives on our collective desire for transformation, offering a seemingly endless array of products and services that claim to unlock our potential.

Yet for all the motivational books, wellness apps, and life coaches promising to help us become our best selves, the data tell a different story. In markets where people spend the most on self-improvement, levels of life satisfaction are close to all-time lows.[443,444] For example, North America, which accounts for 36 percent of the world's self-improvement spending, is experiencing its lowest levels of life satisfaction despite more than twenty years of growth in the category.[444,445,446]

Self-Improvement Spending Relative To Life Satisfaction

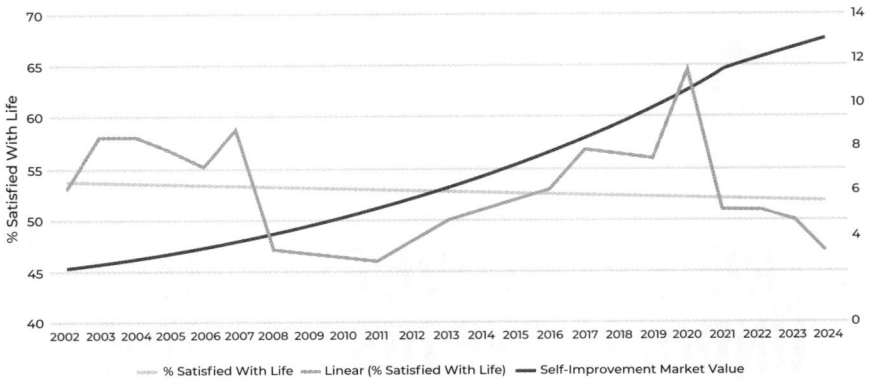

Sources: North American Data based on Gallup, Grand View Research and estimations by Starker, S. (2002)

This paradox exposes an uncomfortable truth: The harder we chase transformation, the more elusive it becomes. The problem lies in the story that the self-improvement movement tells us about success—a story often at odds with the decades of evidence describing what truly sustains human motivation and personal growth.

Self-determination theory—one of the most enduring and extensively researched models in psychology—provides a lens for understanding where self-help has veered off course—and how we may be able to get back on track. At its core, the theory proposes that humans have the following three innate and essential psychological needs:

Autonomy—the need to feel self-directed.

Competence—the need to feel capable and effective.

Relatedness—the need to feel connected to others.

Cumulative insights from years of study reveal a compelling truth: When these fundamental needs are met, we experience greater motivation, engagement, and life satisfaction, laying the groundwork for improved well-being and sustained performance.[447,448,449,450,451,452] However, popular self-improvement narratives and beliefs have distorted the natural drive to satisfy these needs.

Let's explore what this means in practice.

1. THE DISTORTION OF PASSION: "YOU NEED MORE DRIVE"

Conventional self-improvement wisdom often insists that true transformation demands burning passion—a relentless, high-octane drive to pour huge amounts of time and energy into our goals. I agree that passion can be a powerful and effective motivator. Yet in some self-improvement circles, passion is portrayed as autonomy on steroids—an intense inner force propelling us irresistibly toward success. The *hyperoptimizers* and *hustle culture* champions introduced in earlier chapters are fervent advocates of this belief. They contend that to unlock our full potential, we must "go all in," "grind harder," and "make big moves." These notions aren't inherently flawed, but they're framed as one-dimensional. The allegation? If we fall short, it's because we lack the drive.

2. THE DISTORTION OF DISCIPLINE: "YOU NEED MORE SELF-CONTROL"

In the self-improvement world, drive is insufficient. You're expected to pair it with unwavering discipline based on the belief that iron willpower is the key to transformation. The evidence is compelling that self-control is essential.[453] However, too many self-improvement gurus exploit our natural drive for competence—the need to feel capable and effective—and recast it as a requirement to optimize every moment. To be competent, we're told, is to dial in with precise, often all-consuming routines and rituals—usually beginning at 5:00 a.m., ideally earlier, as we explored in chapter 1. The implication? If progress is lacking, you haven't "taken control of yourself."

3. THE DISTORTION OF PERSISTENCE: "YOU NEED MORE GRIT"

Grit—a combination of passion and perseverance toward long-term goals—is the icing on top of the self-improvement cake.[454,455,456] Grit is an admirable quality, but it's been co-opted to suggest that success is simply a matter of pushing hard enough for long enough. This creed is pervasive in *hustle culture,* where excessive work regimes become normalized based on the belief that success is directly proportional to effort and time, leading to seventy-hour weeks or even one-hundred-plus-hour weeks.[457] The inference is that if you didn't experience the transformation you were looking for, you gave up too soon.

4. THE DISTORTION OF SOLITUDE: "YOU NEED MORE SELF-FOCUS"

Self-help narratives often elevate individualism to near mythic status. Take *monk mode,* for example—a self-disciplined monastic life reimagined and repackaged for the TikTok generation. Across social media, thousands, particularly young men, advocate the idea that retreating mentally, physically, and socially can unlock extraordinary personal growth. This philosophy resonates. It's a pushback against hyperconnectivity in our always-on world and taps into a recognition that time alone can be transformative. However, these individualistic approaches often recast self-improvement as a zero-sum game. Prioritizing others or investing in relationships is seen as detrimental to personal progress. The misleading message? If you're struggling and trying to change, double down on self-focus rather than seeking connection.

Simplistic Self-Improvement Fails to Deliver

These distortions reveal a broader trend within the self-improvement industry: reducing complex human behavior to simplistic formulas of willpower, discipline, persistence, and self-reliance. While these qualities can contribute to personal growth, treating them as one-size-fits-all solutions ignores the nuanced ways they manifest in each of us. At its worst, this approach risks amplifying the dissatisfaction and disconnection that lead many to seek self-improvement in the first place.

As we explored in previous chapters, cultivating a shoshin beginner's mind can help us meet this challenge by fostering openness and curiosity, setting the stage for a deeper understanding of the complexity of our motivations, and opening pathways to realize more of our potential.

Beyond the Hype: Sustainable Motivation Requires More than Just Drive

The issue with the *more drive* distortion is its assumption that sustainable motivation springs from the sheer intensity of desire and the relentless application of psychological energy. In reality this approach can sabotage the autonomy and intrinsic motivation essential for lasting change. Research on the dual nature of passion—which can be described as either *harmonious* or obsessive—sheds light on how this dynamic plays out in practice.[458,459]

Ideally, our predominant experience is one of *harmonious passion*—a state where we pursue activities autonomously, driven by a genuine alignment with our values and sense of self. In this mode our motivation stems from enjoyment rather than external pressures or the pursuit of rewards. People with *harmonious passion* approach their work with a sense of autonomy and flexibility, making the process itself rewarding.

Imagine a project manager leading a major initiative at an education tech company. She's committed to her work not only for the outcome—delivering a successful project—but also because she genuinely enjoys the problem-solving and collaboration involved. Her motivation is self-determined and intrinsic; the work itself is satisfying and aligns with her values.

She also experiences extrinsic motivation: She's driven to deliver the project because it contributes to a cause she cares about—developing technology that improves access to education. This reflects *integrated regulation*—the healthiest form of extrinsic motivation—where her effort supports her core values and long-term goals.

At the same time, she feels a sense of control. If unforeseen demands arise, she can step back temporarily without guilt, recognizing that rest and flexibility are integral to sustained performance. Her work is woven naturally into her life, allowing her to feel accomplished and fulfilled without sacrificing her personal life or other priorities.

Harmonious passion fosters positive emotions, a sense of flow, and the pursuit of mastery-oriented goals—where individuals focus on performing at *their* best—leading to improved well-being and performance.[460,461,462]

Obsessive Passion and Perfectionism Sabotage Genuine Fulfillment

Obsessive passion arises when we pursue something because of external pressures rather than freely and autonomously. In this state motivation is driven by outside demands or the lure of rewards, leading to a loss of autonomy and often a relentless, rigid persistence. People who primarily experience *obsessive passion* feel compelled to engage in their pursuits, even when it disrupts other areas of life, making them more susceptible to stress and frustration.

Obsessive passion often goes hand in hand with *perfectionism*—both *self-oriented perfectionism,* which involves holding excessively high personal standards, and *socially prescribed perfectionism*—the belief that others demand perfection from us.[463,464]

Consider a dedicated consultant who takes on a high-stakes project with the initial excitement of delivering value to clients. However, he soon becomes consumed with executing every task flawlessly, sharing every milestone publicly, and pushing through late nights, even when it compromises his health. This is *external regulation*—the least healthy form of extrinsic motivation. Missing a deadline feels like a personal failure, and he worries about colleagues and clients judging him if he's anything short of perfect.

What started as a fulfilling challenge driven by genuine motivation becomes riddled with anxiety. The work shifts from personal growth to an endless loop of "just one more task" as he sacrifices relationships and other commitments to maintain a relentless pace. Research shows that this kind of *obsessive passion* is associated with psychological inflexibility and compulsive work patterns that persist despite negative impacts on health and well-being.[465]

Obsessive passion often leads to poorer or, at best, inconsistent well-being and performance outcomes.[460,461,462,466,467,468,469] Rather than supporting growth, *obsessive passion* fuels rumination—repetitive, unwanted thoughts—and disrupts flow experiences, leaving people caught in cycles of stress and distraction.[461] In work settings *obsessive passion* has also been linked to heightened conflict and increased risk of burnout.[465]

Few of us experience entirely *harmonious* or *obsessive passion*; it's usually a blend of both. Yet with its constant stream of sound bites, clips, and polished personal brands, the self-improvement media landscape increasingly pushes us toward the obsessive side. We're fed a narrative that relentless drive and intensity are the keys to success.

The Paradox of Self-Control: More Is Not Necessarily Better

According to leading psychologists, including the legendary Roy Baumeister, a giant in the world of self-control research, the human capacity to exert self-control—often called self-regulation, self-discipline, or willpower—is "arguably one of the most powerful and beneficial adaptations of the human psyche."[470]

The self-improvement industry has a love affair with self-control. Browse any self-help bestseller list and you'll find countless promises that mastering self-control is the key to unlocking your best life. The narrative is simple and seductive: Successful people exhibit more self-control, so developing more of it should make us more successful, too. Research does lend weight to this idea, showing that high levels of *trait self-control* predict better health, greater wealth, and stronger relationships.[471,472] But this "more is better" view of self-control only tells half the story.[473]

Self-control operates at two levels: *trait self-control* (a stable personality trait) and *state self-control* (the ability to resist temptation in the moment). While high trait self-control consistently aligns with positive life outcomes, the impact of state self-control on success is far more complex, but this nuance is often lost in simplistic self-help stories.[474]

Relying heavily on momentary state self-control—the gritted-teeth resistance to temptation championed in self-help circles—can backfire. When we use sheer willpower to suppress our desires repeatedly, we often fall into the *triangular relapse pattern* that I introduced in chapter 1.

Initiation: Motivation peaks, driving ambitious goals and new routines.

Maintenance: Initial enthusiasm fades, making it harder to sustain effort.

Setback: Motivation declines further, leading to a return to old habits, often accompanied by frustration and guilt.

This pattern is all too familiar, and when it occurs, people often berate themselves, assuming they simply lack willpower. Observing *hyperoptimizer* icons—those who appear to rise at 5:00 a.m., adhere to rigid routines and juggle a dazzling list of self-improvement protocols—only worsens the sense of inadequacy.

But here lies the misconception: Those who appear to possess ironclad self-control aren't constantly battling temptation.[473] Instead, they've crafted their world to minimize the need for willpower. Rather than wrestling with resistance, they design lives that sidestep it.

When Perfect Routines Meet Real Life: The Limits of Life Design

Designing our lives and environments to make desired behaviors easier can be a very effective strategy for sustaining change. However, taken to an extreme, this approach can also begin to limit our freedom, diminishing the sense of autonomy and competence it was meant to enhance—especially when perfectly crafted routines encounter the unpredictability of real life.

Consider Marie Kondo, the queen of decluttering and minimalism, who rose to fame promoting the idea that a perfectly ordered environment sparks joy and fosters a well-organized life. Recently, however, Kondo admitted that she found it impossible to maintain her famously pristine home after having children. The rigid system that once provided calm became a source of stress, prompting her to give up on constant tidying to spend more time with her family.[475]

Life design can work wonderfully when everything is under control, but when life becomes chaotic—as it inevitably does—these systems often crumble under new pressures. Kondo's ability to adapt demonstrates admirable psychological flexibility and a willingness to do what was best for herself and her family, regardless of followers' expectations. Unfortunately, many struggle to be as ready or able to change.

Beware the Costs of Very High Self-Control

There's also a bleaker side to self-control that the self-improvement movement rarely acknowledges. For example, research has revealed that when older adults reflect on their lives, excessive self-control—choosing work over pleasure, duty over joy—is often a source of deep regret.[476] The benefits of very high *trait self-control* may come at the cost of missed opportunities and experiences that arise from being open to deviation from strict routines.[474]

Consider the example of a high-achieving professional who, throughout their career, consistently chose work over leisure and personal relationships. Driven by a strong sense of duty and high self-control, they prioritized career milestones over family gatherings, vacations, and even small moments of relaxation. Decades later, they find themselves financially secure but often reflecting with regret on the relationships they missed and the experiences they set aside in favor of work.

Watch Out for Puritanical Bias

Finally, the self-improvement industry's obsession with self-control often places too much emphasis on individual responsibility, overlooking broader influences. Take obesity: It's frequently framed as a failure of self-control, where overeating is seen as a personal flaw. This view ignores key factors such as access to affordable, nutritious foods versus the prevalence of cheap, calorie-dense processed options that promote overeating. This oversimplification, known as *puritanical bias,* reduces complex issues to personal shortcomings while dismissing critical environmental and socio-economic factors.[27]

The takeaway *is not* that self-control or personal accountability lack value but that the link between self-control and self-improvement is more nuanced than the self-help industry suggests. It's not that we need more self-control; we need to use the self-control we have more strategically.

Rethinking Grit: This "Secret to Success" May Not Be So Malleable

Grit—a fusion of passion and perseverance directed toward long-term goals—has long been celebrated as a self-improvement magic bullet. We're told that passion fuels drive, self-control enforces discipline, and grit (combining both) is the secret ingredient that guarantees we'll prevail.[477]

However, emerging research suggests that the story may be more complex and that grit may not be as malleable as initially thought. The critic's central argument is that grit functions more like a stable *trait* than a flexible *state*, challenging the idea that it can be significantly improved.

States refer to how we feel or behave in the moment. For example, you might feel motivated before the kickoff of a big project. States can often easily shift through interventions—actions and programs designed to create positive changes or improvements. For instance, you could improve motivation with goal setting and progress tracking. Imagine states as visiting cousins—they pop in and out depending on the situation—that are temporary and changeable.

Traits are more like siblings—steadfast, familiar, and reliable. Traits include personality characteristics such as being generally agreeable or extroverted. While it's not impossible to change them, traits tend to be stable, enduring, and resistant to modification.

When researchers dove deeper to analyze the characteristics of grit, they noticed that it was closely correlated with *trait self-control*, which relates to a person's relatively stable predisposition to manage their impulses and make decisions that align with their goals.[455,478] From a statistical point of view, grit also looked a lot like *conscientiousness*—the personality trait associated with reliability, organization, and responsibility.[455,478] Further, researchers noted a strong genetic basis for conscientiousness and *perseverance of effort*—a core component of grit. This observation suggests that the same genetic factors may influence both these stable traits and grit.[455,478] Together, these findings point to grit having a largely stable, heritable component, making it resistant to change. In short it looks like grit might be a close sibling rather than a visiting cousin.

This insight has significant implications for self-improvement. If grit is essentially a stable trait, it may be far less changeable and, therefore, less amenable to improvement by effort and interventions than the self-help industry claims.

Grit's Predictive Power Is in Question

Further, the distinctiveness of grit as a predictor of success has increasingly come into question, particularly because of its overlap with other well-established psychological frameworks. Critics argue that for grit to warrant focused development, it must offer predictive power above and beyond qualities such as *self-control* or *conscientiousness*. In other words, for grit to be worth improving, higher grit levels should lead to better outcomes that cannot be attributed to other traits.

Supporting the critics' view, studies reveal that, when predicting academic performance, grit's key component, *perseverance of effort*, does not outperform the stable trait of *effort regulation*—a quality reflecting consistent capacity for self-discipline and sustained effort.[479] Similarly, research has shown that grit fails to uniquely predict GPA, a standard measure of academic success, when *conscientiousness*—a stable personality trait—is accounted for.[480] These findings suggest that grit may add little unique value, challenging its status as a stand-alone factor in achieving long-term success.

It's important to note that counternarratives argue for the distinctiveness of *grit* and contend that it can be developed and improved.[477] However, the weight of evidence pointing to its stability and genetic basis emphasizes that the self-improvement mantra of "you just need more grit" is oversimplistic and potentially misleading.

High Grit May Increase Susceptibility to Cognitive Biases

Even if we can improve grit, there are times when pivoting, shifting interests, or reassessing goals is the wiser path.[456,481,482] Overusing grit is like driving on the highway without noticing you've missed your exit—continuing at full speed, pedal to the metal, yet moving further from your intended destination. For example, in sports, practice makes permanent, not necessarily perfect. Repeating flawed patterns only reinforces mistakes. In the workplace misplaced grit can become *costly perseverance*, where individuals double down on failing efforts.[483]

Research also suggests that people high in grit may be more vulnerable to some *cognitive biases*—mental shortcuts that shape our perceptions and decisions. This includes greater susceptibility to the *sunk cost fallacy*, which leads people to continue investing in a decision or project simply because they've already devoted significant resources despite evidence that it may no longer be beneficial.[483] For example, in one study, over half of aspiring inventors continued investing time, effort, and money in doomed projects despite expert advice to stop.[484]

High grit can also heighten people's susceptibility to *fading affect bias*.[485] This bias has two key effects. First, over time, positive memories retain their emotional impact more vividly than negative ones, making people more likely to recall past successes and enjoyable moments with clarity and warmth while their struggles fade into the background. Second, *fading affect bias* alters how negative experiences are remembered: The memory of unpleasant events softens more than is typical, and in hindsight they often take on a rosier hue than they originally had. While this bias can be adaptive—helping maintain resilience and a positive outlook—it also risks blurring self-awareness, making it harder to accurately assess past challenges or recognize when grit may lead them astray.

These tendencies can blend with other cognitive biases to which we are all vulnerable to some extent, creating a powerful and potentially risky combination. For example, the *endowment effect* can lead us to overvalue something simply because we own it, making it harder to let go even when it's no longer beneficial. *Status quo bias* describes our preference for keeping things the same over making changes, often because of fear of the unknown or the comfort of familiarity. *Loss aversion* can make us fear losses more than gains of equal value.

Let's make this practical. Imagine Erica, a former elite athlete turned tech founder whose start-up is sending clear distress signals. Market feedback suggests her product has missed its mark, and financial reserves are depleting rapidly. Yet she remains anchored to her original vision with the tenacity that once made her a formidable competitor. "Winners never quit" isn't just her mantra—it's a core part of her identity. However, this character strength of *perseverance* is being hijacked by cognitive biases:

1. Her brain's *sunk cost calculator* keeps a meticulous ledger of every hour and dollar invested in the existing path, making it harder to pivot or walk away.
2. The *endowment effect* causes her to attribute a much higher value to the business than is justifiable with objective metrics, making it difficult to secure more funding from investors with more conservative valuations.
3. *Status quo bias* wraps her existing strategy in a comfortable blanket of familiarity.
4. *Loss aversion* amplifies every potential downside of changing course while minimizing the perceived value of opportunities.
5. The *fading affect bias* acts as a selective filter for her memories, brightening past victories while softening the sharp edges of setbacks.

Together, these biases cloud Erica's perspective, anchoring her to a draining path and blinding her to the opportunity costs. What started as grit has turned into an emotional and cognitive trap. But these risks and biases don't just apply to entrepreneurs; we're all vulnerable to some extent.

How Long Does It Take to Build a Habit?

Beyond keeping us on paths that may no longer serve us, the belief that success is simply a matter of *sticking with it* can also warp our expectations about how quickly we can change behavior and build habits. Many people latch onto so-called magic numbers—like the widely circulated claim that it takes twenty-one days to form a new habit.

This notion originates from observations of plastic surgery patients who seemed to adapt to their new looks within twenty-one days.[486,487] Yet despite its narrow context, this timeframe has been widely generalized, applied far beyond appearance adjustment to nearly any habit change.

Other studies suggest a different timeline, finding that it takes an average of sixty-six days for a behavior to become second nature.[488] However, more recent research indicates that there is no universal timeline for transformation.[489] An analysis of data from twenty studies found that habits related to exercise, hydration, or following a healthy diet took, on average, 106 to 154 days to establish. At an individual level, the researchers observed that habits could form in as few as four days or as long as 335 days. These findings highlight that the time required to form a habit can vary widely, influenced by factors such as the complexity of the behavior, its frequency of repetition, the nature of its rewards, and individual differences.[490]

Exploding the Myth of the 10,000-Hour Rule

It's not just habit change. The self-improvement world loves almost any kind of magic number. You've probably heard of the famed *10,000-hour rule*—the idea that mastering a complex skill or becoming expert in a field requires 10,000 hours of practice.[491] However, the rule misrepresented the research on which it was based. The original study found that elite musicians averaged over 10,000 hours of practice by age twenty, but this was simply an average, not a finish line for expertise.[492] In fact, only about half of the top violinists had reached this milestone.

Anders Ericsson, the acclaimed scientist behind the original studies, was notably critical of how his work was popularized as a one-size-fits-all pathway. Alarmed by the media's oversimplifications, he even penned an open letter, "The Danger of Delegating Education to Journalists," to debunk the myth of the 10,000-hour rule.[493]

The rule's emphasis on time alone overlooks a critical aspect: practice quality. Not all practice contributes equally to improvement. High-quality, focused, *deliberate practice*—where feedback and continual adjustments are central—matters far more than mere hours. But even deliberate practice isn't a guarantee of success. Studies show that deliberate practice explains only part of skill variation: 26 percent in chess, 21 percent in music, 18 percent in sports, and less than 1 percent in the workplace.[494,495] These findings highlight that other factors—innate talent, learning environment, and even luck—play key roles in shaping expertise.

The 10,000-hour rule distorts our innate desire for competence by turning mastery into a rigid formula, suggesting that anyone can achieve expertise with enough time and sheer effort. True *competence*, however, is about feeling capable and effective through meaningful, self-directed activities aligned with our values and interests. Moreover, this one-size-fits-all approach can undermine *autonomy*, nudging people into mechanical routines focused on hitting milestones rather than cultivating genuine growth.

Ultimately, while persistence matters, this oversimplified view of grit has led to an unthinking form of stubborn persistence, divorced from our genuine needs and capabilities. We need to work smarter—not just harder, faster, and longer—by paying attention to the map and our destination rather than fixating on the accelerator pedal.

We also need to challenge the notion that the journey is best made alone.

Too Much Self-Reliance Is Self-Limiting

The allure of the lone warrior on a quest for self-mastery runs deep in cultural mythology. From ancient ascetics to modern *monk mode* influencers, we're drawn to narratives of radical self-reliance and isolation as paths to personal growth. These accounts have some truth. Time alone can be transformative.

However, hyperindividualistic philosophies overlook a critical aspect of how human beings grow and thrive. No one transforms and reaches their potential in a vacuum. We thrive when we feel self-directed, capable, *and* connected.[448,449]

Autonomy—the need to feel self-directed—is often misunderstood as opposing community or relatedness, but that's not true.[4-7] *Autonomy* is about having the freedom to make choices that feel true to yourself, but those choices could be independent or aligned with a community.

For example, imagine an analyst who decides to stay late at work on a big project. They're not staying because they fear their boss's reaction if they leave but because they genuinely value the work and want to contribute to the team's success. They act independently in terms of their choice, but their decision is also deeply rooted in their commitment to the group. Research supports this idea, showing that autonomy can strengthen relationships, like with family or friends, rather than pulling people apart.[496,497,498] In short, the fundamental needs of *autonomy*, *competence*, and *relatedness* are not in competition—they're complementary.

It's time to let go of the myths of rugged individualism. While *monk mode* may trend on social media, the reality on the ground tells a different story. Social isolation has become a pressing issue.

Loneliness Is on the Rise

Adult loneliness has steadily risen since the 1970s.[499] One in ten people say they have no close friends.[500] Half of adults report feeling lonely, with some of the highest rates among young adults—contrary to the popular image of loneliness as primarily an elderly person's burden.[501] Remote working may be exacerbating this trend. Nearly three-quarters of workers under thirty-five feel their colleagues are growing more distant, and over 80 percent worry about the loneliness of long-term remote work.[502]

The consequences are far-reaching. Loneliness and social isolation increase the risk of premature death by 26 to 29 percent.[501] They're associated with a 29 percent higher risk of heart disease and a 32 percent higher risk of stroke.[501] Adults who frequently feel lonely are more than twice as likely to develop depression compared with those who rarely or never experience loneliness.[503] A review of sixty-three studies found that loneliness and social isolation in children and adolescents significantly increase their risk of depression and anxiety, with effects that can persist for up to nine years.[504] It's also notable that research into entrepreneurs' mental health indicates that a combination of obsessive passion and social isolation is a leading factor contributing to burnout.[505] The evidence is clear—loneliness isn't just a fleeting emotion; it also has lasting impacts on mental health across all age groups.

But if isolation poses such serious risks, could actively fostering connection and investment in other people be part of the solution?

Self-Care Should Not Be Selfish

One of the most persistent self-improvement myths is that personal growth and helping others are in competition, leading many people to become increasingly self-focused in the name of *working on themselves*. Influencers assure us that taking time out for self-care is not selfish— and, to a point, they're right. Everyone needs time alone to recharge. But when self-care becomes self-absorption, it misses the mark entirely. This narrow, zero-sum view ignores compelling research showing that social connection and contributing to others don't detract from personal growth; they enhance it.

A fascinating series of studies found that beneficence—the feeling of making a positive impact on others—is a significant predictor of well-being.[450] Moreover, the link between prosocial behavior (actions intended to benefit others) and well-being is largely driven by increased feelings of autonomy, competence, and relatedness.[450] In other words helping others boosts all our most fundamental and vital human needs.

Consider someone volunteering at a local food bank. By choosing to help, they experience a sense of agency (autonomy). As they grow more skilled at organizing donations, they feel effective and capable (competence). And by working with others to support those in need, they feel a deeper bond with their community (relatedness). These experiences collectively enhance their well-being, while their actions also benefit the recipients.

This shouldn't come as a surprise. As inherently social beings, humans evolved to thrive in community. Meeting our need for relatedness predicts a wide range of positive outcomes, from intrinsic motivation to resilience in the face of challenges to the internalization of healthy behaviors—adopting positive habits or practices in a way that makes them feel natural, self-driven, and integrated into our identity.[447,449]

True personal growth doesn't force a choice between self and others. Real transformation seldom happens in isolation. The deepest growth occurs when we invest in ourselves while contributing to others, grounded in relationships that satisfy our core needs for autonomy, competence, and connection.

Next, we'll explore how we can find a path that avoids extremes and cuts through the oversimplification of self-help clichés. We'll begin by tackling the distortion of passion and the myth that we simply need more drive.

Foster Harmonious Passion: Stay on the Healthy Side of Drive

Obsessive passion can infiltrate nearly any goal or area of self-improvement, locking us into rigid persistence rather than healthy drive. So how can we improve our chances of staying on the healthier, *harmonious* side of passion? Practical studies on cultivating *harmonious passion* are limited, but research into the *dualistic model* of passion suggests a few strategies, starting with the following two steps:

> **Acknowledge Duality:** Understanding that most of us experience both *harmonious* and *obsessive passion* to varying degrees is the first step to nurturing one more than the other.

> **Assess Your Baseline:** Measuring your *harmonious* and *obsessive passion* balance, such as by using the following assessment scale, can help you identify areas to focus on.[459]

In the context of a personal or professional activity you are passionate about, answer each item on a 7-point scale, ranging from 1 (*I do not agree at all*) to 7 (*I completely agree*).

PART 1							
This activity allows me to live a variety of experiences.	1	2	3	4	5	6	7
The new things that I discover with this activity allow me to appreciate it even more.	1	2	3	4	5	6	7
This activity allows me to live memorable experiences.	1	2	3	4	5	6	7
This activity reflects the qualities I like about myself.	1	2	3	4	5	6	7
This activity is in harmony with the other activities in my life.	1	2	3	4	5	6	7
For me, it is a passion that I still manage to control.	1	2	3	4	5	6	7
I am completely taken with this activity.	1	2	3	4	5	6	7
PART 1 AVERAGE SCORE:							

PART 2							
I cannot live without it.	1	2	3	4	5	6	7
The urge is so strong. I can't help myself from doing this activity.	1	2	3	4	5	6	7
I have difficulty imagining my life without this activity.	1	2	3	4	5	6	7
I am emotionally dependent on this activity.	1	2	3	4	5	6	7
I have a tough time controlling my need to do this activity.	1	2	3	4	5	6	7
I have almost an obsessive feeling for this activity.	1	2	3	4	5	6	7
My mood depends on me being able to do this activity.	1	2	3	4	5	6	7
PART 2 AVERAGE SCORE:							

Calculate your average score for parts 1 and 2 separately. The average rating for part 1 provides your *harmonious passion* score. The average score for part 2 represents your *obsessive passion* score. Compare the relationship between the two scores.

Aim for a Net-Harmonious score by intentionally developing practices that support *harmonious passion* while minimizing factors that may shift you toward *obsessive passion*.

Use Your Signature Strengths to Cultivate Harmonious Passion

Research indicates that one of the most effective ways to cultivate *harmonious passion* is by identifying and applying our *signature strengths*—the top-ranked character strengths introduced in chapter 7.[506]

Start by identifying your *signature strengths*. As mentioned in chapter 7, you can do this by taking the free, scientifically validated character strengths assessment from the VIA Institute on Character.[441] Once you've identified your strengths, set aside some time to complete the following exercise.

When Are You at Your Best? Describe a time when you were working at your best. What did it look like, and how did you apply your signature strengths? Reflect on how you felt before, during, and after using these strengths.

Put Your Strengths into Action. Think of a way to use two of your signature strengths in new ways during the next two weeks.

Acknowledge the Impact. Reflect on the positive outcomes that arose from using your *signature strengths* and consider how they influenced your work or personal growth.

When repeated over time, even this short activity could put you on the right track to a more harmonious relationship with passion.

Counter Perfectionism with Self-Compassion

If you lean toward *obsessive passion,* actively countering the perfectionism that often accompanies it may also be helpful.[463] If this resonates, know that you're not alone. Over the past thirty-five years, *socially prescribed perfectionism*—the belief that others expect us to be flawless—has surged by 33 percent, while self-oriented perfectionism, where we impose excessively high standards on ourselves, has increased by 10 percent.[507] Fortunately, there's an effective antidote—practicing self-compassion.[508]

The following are the three components that characterize self-compassion:

Self-Kindness: Treat yourself with the same kindness you'd extend to a friend. When faced with setbacks, try to swap harsh criticism for understanding and support, recognizing that mistakes are part of growth.

Common Humanity: Remember, suffering and struggle are universal. When things go wrong, it's not just you—everyone faces challenges. Embracing this shared experience eases isolation and can foster resilience.

Mindfulness: Take a nonjudgmental look at your emotions. Consider how you could adopt a shoshin mindset, observing your emotions with curiosity and freeing yourself from the pressure of needing to have all the answers.

Think of self-compassion as a psychological shock absorber. When perfectionists hit the inevitable bumps of failure or perceived inadequacy, those with high self-compassion don't crash nearly as hard. The research shows that while perfectionists typically spiral when things aren't just right, this tendency significantly weakens when they practice self-compassion. Recent research has even revealed that people who practice self-compassion lower their risk of cardiovascular disease. The effect was independent of blood pressure, insulin resistance, and cholesterol levels, supporting the notion that self-compassion is responsible for the benefits.[509]

Rethinking Willpower: Self-Control Is Not a Limited Resource

While we're on the topic of blood pressure and cholesterol, I'm sure we can all relate to the experience of staring down a slice of chocolate cake while reciting willpower mantras. On second thought, perhaps that's just me, but regardless of whether your vice is sweet foods, social media scrolling, or something else, the popular self-improvement solution is the same: "You need more self-control." But what if that advice misses the mark? What if the real key to self-control lies not in having more of it but in using it differently?

For years we've been told that self-control functions like a fuel tank, slowly draining as we navigate temptations, challenges, and daily obligations.[510] According to this *ego depletion theory,* each act of restraint—saying no to dessert, forcing yourself to exercise, staying focused on work—draws from a limited reservoir of self-control. And when that reservoir is empty, the theory goes, we're bound to succumb to temptation. This perspective implies that our resistance is, at best, temporary and that giving in is an inevitable outcome once our willpower is used up. But more recent research paints a very different picture.

Rather than behaving like a dwindling fuel supply, self-control may be more accurately described as a highly adaptive decision-making process—one that evaluates options based on perceived value rather than sheer stamina.[511,512] When people give in after a long day of exerting self-control, it's often not because they're out of willpower; it's because they've made a real-time assessment that the effort isn't worth it.

Consider this: Have you ever felt too tired to tackle the laundry but suddenly found the energy when an old friend suggested meeting up or seen a student seemingly exhausted from studying instantly rally when a party invitation arrives? These scenarios expose a flaw in the fuel tank view of willpower. What appears to be depleted self-control often reflects a reorientation of priorities. The momentary value of the task has shifted.

The Real Question: How Can We Align Values and Behaviors?

Far from being a finite resource, self-control is a continual reassessment of what's worth our effort, guiding us to recalibrate in real time based on what matters most.

This reframing has far-reaching implications. Instead of asking, "How can I be more self-controlled?" we might do better to ask, "How can I better align my values with my behaviors?" Research shows that when people truly value a goal—when it resonates as meaningful rather than just obligatory—they display a remarkable capacity for sustained self-control.[474,513]

This implication isn't that self-control is boundless but rather that it's tied to our motivational state more than to any finite internal reserve. Trying to build greater reserves of willpower misses the core issue. The real opportunity lies in designing our environments and choices so that our goals and immediate actions align more naturally.

This shifts the focus from resistance to redesign. Rather than constantly working to *strengthen* willpower, we can focus on making desired behaviors inherently more rewarding and reducing the allure of temptations.

As mentioned earlier in this chapter, people with high self-control use less of it in their daily lives.[473] Rather than constantly battling temptation, they've found ways to make good choices more automatic and aligned with their values and bad choices less available.

How to Translate Good Intentions into Action

So how do we put this insight into practice? You can begin by experimenting with the following steps:

Reflect on Why the Behavior Matters: Most people approach change by focusing on what they *should* do. But shoulds are notoriously weak motivators. Instead, connect your desired behavior to what truly matters to you.[514,515] Why exercise? Perhaps it's about having the energy to be fully present with your family. Why save money? Maybe it's about creating future freedom and security. When actions align with authentic values, they shift from burdensome obligations to meaningful choices that serve your deeper purpose.

Start Small and Specific: Habits demand much less mental effort to sustain once ingrained.[473] The biggest challenge is often the first step. Begin by establishing a *minimum viable action*—the smallest meaningful step toward your goal. This can help overcome inertia by reducing the threshold for getting started. For example, if you were aiming to build a habit of exercising daily, you could begin by setting a baseline of ten push-ups. This seemingly insignificant commitment lowers the threshold for getting started, making it more likely that you will string together sessions and establish a consistent routine.

Engineer Your Environment: Instead of using your self-control to overcome frustrations, resist temptations, and act, shape your surroundings to make good choices the most obvious and temptations less visible. For instance, anticipate friction points that could derail new habits. If you were trying to establish an exercise routine, you could commit to laying out your workout clothes the night before and plan your session in advance. If you're tempted to lie in bed scrolling on your phone in the morning, get an alarm clock and leave your phone in another room. Rather than waiting until you feel like working out, where possible, set a consistent time to exercise.

Establish Goals Based on Ranges: Setting a specific numerical goal, like losing exactly two pounds per week or making precisely twenty sales calls per day, might seem logical, but research indicates it may be counterproductive.[516] Instead, aim for a range: one to three pounds or eighteen to twenty-two calls. Why? Because ranges give you the best of both worlds: The lower number feels attainable, preventing discouragement, while the upper number provides an exciting challenge. Studies show that people who set a range of goals are significantly more likely to stick with their efforts in the long term. The key is that it taps into two crucial motivational factors: the satisfaction of reaching an achievable minimum and the thrill of potentially hitting an ambitious maximum.

Focus on the Process: When setting goals, we tend to fixate on the outcome—the final achievement we hope to reach. But neuroscientific insights suggest a different approach: self-propagating goals.[514,515,517,518] In this model each small achievement naturally leads to the next, creating a sustainable cycle of motivation. Breaking goals into smaller, achievable steps releases dopamine—a neurochemical reward that reinforces each action and keeps the drive alive, making the process itself rewarding rather than hinging on a distant end point. Research underscores that process goals, which center on smaller actions within our control, are over fifteen times more effective in driving success than outcome goals that depend on external factors.[519] The real challenge in goal attainment often emerges when motivation dips or the goal feels too far off. Creating process goals with clear, measurable steps can help overcome these dips and support more consistent progress. For instance, consider a professional aiming for a promotion by year-end—a classic outcome goal dependent on external decisions. By reframing this into process goals such as "complete one major project each quarter" and "hold monthly check-ins with my manager," the focus shifts to actionable, controllable steps that steadily build momentum toward the larger aim.

Aim for Progress, Not Perfection: Perhaps most importantly, remind yourself that no habit formation process or behavior change initiative will unfold seamlessly. Be mindful that rigid all-or-nothing mindsets often backfire.[481] In contrast, aiming for continuous progress rather than flawless outcomes is more likely to lead to satisfaction and greater resilience in the face of unexpected twists and turns.[517,518] Once again, practicing *self-compassion*—treating yourself with kindness rather than harsh judgment in the face of failure—can help you stay committed to your goals while reducing the likelihood of giving up entirely when things don't go as planned. Setbacks become learning experiences rather than personal failings.

Think of self-control not as a rigid shield to fend off every temptation but as a strategic adviser guiding you to avoid unnecessary battles. Perfection isn't the goal—habits are built through consistency over time, not flawlessness. It's okay to stumble, miss a day, or even break routine entirely;

these moments don't define your progress. However, we also need to recognize when a struggle is worth the effort and when it's wiser to step back and recalibrate.

We Can't Eliminate Cognitive Biases, but We Can Work Around Them

Whether or not you fully buy into the concept of grit and its potential for improvement, there's no denying that combining *passion* with *perseverance* can be a powerful formula. However, to harness grit effectively, it must be tempered with self-awareness and adaptability—qualities that help us recognize when a change in direction is needed.[456] This is where *cognitive reappraisal*—the mental skill of reinterpreting a situation—can create space to pause, assess our path, and identify where cognitive biases might cloud our judgment.[520]

Consider revisiting the reappraisal techniques from chapter 7 on rethinking stress and apply them to grit. Use them to look closely at both empowering aspects and potential pitfalls. You can also reexamine the character strengths framework in the previous chapter and reflect on how you can use the *tempering effect*—deliberately engaging a balancing strength such as *prudence*, which involves careful planning, foresight, and the ability to weigh risks and benefits—when you notice you're overusing a strength such as *perseverance*.

We can't eliminate cognitive biases—they are deeply rooted in the way our brains process information. However, we can learn to recognize and navigate around them. Think of cognitive biases such as gravity—invisible forces that pull us back into familiar thought patterns. But with the right insights and tools, we can defy these forces, lifting ourselves above their influence and choosing paths aligned with values rather than being tethered to a trajectory that no longer serves us. *Strategic disengagement* represents one such tool, providing a structured approach to decision-making that can help us sidestep the pitfalls of maladaptive mental shortcuts.

Strategic Disengagement: Ensure Perseverance Serves Rather Than Sabotages

Strategic disengagement helps us stay aligned with our values by prompting us to plan our responses in advance—ideally when we're calm and emotionally regulated. This approach makes us less vulnerable to cognitive biases, which often intensify under stress and urgency. Think of strategic disengagement as a buffer between impulse and action, allowing us to respond thoughtfully rather than reactively. Here are five steps to put this theory into practice:

Identify High-Risk Situations: Pinpoint scenarios where you're prone to react impulsively or where cognitive biases may cloud your judgment.

Establish Kill Criteria: This concept, introduced by Annie Duke, a former professional poker player, describes the clear signals that indicate when it's time to quit or pivot a project.[521] Start by carrying out a *premortem*—a planning exercise to anticipate potential pitfalls. Next, establish indicators, such as market shifts or priority changes, which will trigger a pivot or stoppage. This approach helps circumvent the *sunk cost fallacy*—our tendency to persist solely because of past investments—and make more rational decisions.

Plan Your Responses: Outline specific, values-driven responses you can turn to in high-stress moments. For example, preparing cognitive reappraisals—reinterpretations of situations—in advance of high-stakes moments can be helpful. Identify your most common cognitive biases and craft alternative narratives to reshape your perspective in line with your values. For example, the *sunk cost fallacy* ("I've already put so much into this; I can't stop now") could be reframed as "Every investment teaches us something. I can shift direction if that best serves the business."

Pause to Seek External Perspectives: Our cognitive biases often blind us to the reality of our situations, but trusted advisors with our long-term interests can provide crucial objectivity. For example, they can counter the *endowment effect* by helping us focus on its true value rather than personal attachment. Advisors can also help us distinguish between productive struggle and destructive suffering.

Consider appointing a personal board of advisors and set a consistent schedule to check in with them.

Recalculate Expected Value: Revisit the *expected value* decision-making equation that I introduced at the end of chapter 1: *Expected Value = (Potential Benefits × Probability of Benefits) - (Potential Risks × Probability of Risks) - Implementation Costs.* Use it to evaluate whether your current path consistently offers more benefits than downsides across different scenarios.

Once again, to make this practical, let's rewind and watch how the same scenario unfolds when Erica, the former athlete turned tech entrepreneur, applies *strategic disengagement.*

1. Anticipating the Cognitive Storm

Early in her journey, Erica recognizes her athlete's mindset could become a double-edged sword. She maps out specific scenarios where her competitive drive might override rational decision-making. "My greatest strength in sports was never giving up," she reflects. "But in business, knowing when to pivot is equally crucial."

2. Setting Clear Kill Switches

Working with her advisors, Erica establishes concrete metrics that would trigger a strategic review.

- Three consecutive quarters of declining user engagement.
- Cash runway dropping below six months without a clear path to profitability.
- Market feedback consistently pointing to fundamental product market fit issues.

These aren't just numbers—they're also *cognitive circuit breakers* designed to override emotional decision-making when necessary.

3. Reframing the Narrative

Erica develops a new mental playbook. When the *sunk cost fallacy* whispers, "You've invested too much to quit," she counters with "Every dollar spent has purchased valuable market intelligence." Her athlete's mindset of "winners never quit" evolves into "champions make strategic adjustments."

4. Building an Objectivity Shield

She assembles a personal board of advisors—including a seasoned entrepreneur, a market analyst, and a former mentor from her athletic days. They meet quarterly, providing the emotional distance needed to see her venture clearly. When the *endowment effect* clouds her judgment, their external perspective helps restore clarity.

5. Running the Numbers

Rather than relying on gut feelings, Erica regularly updates her expected value calculations, weighing potential benefits against risks and implementation costs across multiple scenarios. This quantitative approach helps cut through the emotional fog of decision-making.

When market signals turn negative, and her kill criteria are triggered, Erica doesn't see it as defeat. Instead, she recognizes an opportunity to demonstrate true entrepreneurial athleticism—the ability to pivot strategically.

Develop the Courage to Change Course in Light of New Evidence

What separates this version of Erica from her counterpart isn't intelligence or capability—it's the recognition that our minds, brilliant as they are, come with cognitive blind spots. Strategic disengagement isn't about dampening our passionate pursuit of goals; it's about ensuring that passion serves rather than sabotages our success.

In the end, the greatest demonstration of grit might not be persisting against all odds but having the sense of *autonomy*, *competence*, and *courage* to change course when the evidence demands it. As Erica discovered, sometimes the most powerful move in our performance playbook is knowing when to quit.

The Most Effective Self-Improvement Is Not Self-Centered

As I mentioned earlier, entrepreneurs' obsessive passion can contribute to a higher risk of burnout, but social isolation is also a key contributor—something we are all vulnerable to.[505]

Despite what some self-improvement philosophies may imply, our connections to others and contributions to their lives aren't distractions from personal growth—they're essential to it. Our *relatedness*—feeling connected to others—is a core human need that plays a significant role in our well-being and development.[448,449]

However, there's a risk that even relationships can be subsumed into overoptimization, where connection becomes something to be achieved or collected, reducing relationships to transactions. But the answer to isolation isn't about increasing the number of friends or social interactions; it's about creating environments where genuine connections can emerge naturally.

Research points to some practical ways to cultivate these meaningful connections.[501]

Make It Intentional: Set aside dedicated, distraction-free time each day to connect with friends or family. Put your phone away during meals and important conversations.

Quality over Quantity: Strengthening existing relationships can have a greater impact than expanding your social circle. Even a few close, trusted confidants can provide significant support and reduce feelings of loneliness.

Authentic Self-Expression: Instead of aiming to be more social, focus on spaces where you can genuinely express yourself. This might mean joining groups or activities aligned with your interests or values, where authenticity can come naturally.

Small Actions Matter: A brief, genuine interaction can positively influence both you and the person you're connecting with. For instance, recent research indicates that just one quality conversation with a friend each day could significantly boost well-being.[522]

Community Engagement: Contributing to the community—through volunteering, joining local organizations, or participating in neighborhood activities—creates organic opportunities to connect while meeting our innate need for relatedness.

The fifth approach—*community* engagement—highlights another powerful driver of well-being that is even more antithetical to self-centered development: beneficence (the sense of making a positive difference in others' lives). Beneficence isn't just a lofty ideal; it's also a vital component in personal development and life satisfaction.[450] When people feel they're positively influencing others, they report higher levels of energy, authentic motivation, and a stronger alignment with their core values.[523] Research also shows that people who pursue intrinsic goals such as community contribution and meaningful relationships experience greater well-being than those chasing extrinsic goals such as wealth and status.[450,523] By helping others, we help ourselves grow.

True self-improvement isn't self-centered—it's self-expanding.

So perhaps it's time to retire the image of self-improvement as a solitary journey of individual optimization. Instead, we might think of it as more like tending a garden—one where our autonomy and growth are inextricably linked to the success of those around us. By nurturing our relationships and finding ways to contribute to others' lives, we create the conditions for everyone to thrive.

CHAPTER 8 REVIEW

In this chapter we explored why self-improvement efforts often fail despite good intentions. We examined how self-determination theory's core needs—*autonomy, competence,* and *relatedness*—get distorted by common self-improvement narratives and discovered more sustainable approaches to personal growth.

KEY INSIGHTS

COMMON SELF-IMPROVEMENT DISTORTIONS

- **Passion:** "You need more drive."
- **Discipline:** "You need more self-control."
- **Persistence:** "You need more grit."
- **Solitude:** "You need more self-focus."

UNDERSTANDING PASSION TYPES

- **Harmonious passion:** autonomous, flexible pursuit of activities.
- **Obsessive passion:** rigid, compulsive engagement.
- Most experience both types to varying degrees.
- Balance is needed for sustainable motivation.

SELF-CONTROL REALITIES

- Not a limited resource to be depleted.
- More about value-based decision-making.
- High self-control users often avoid temptation.
- Environmental design matters more than willpower.

SOCIAL CONNECTION IMPACT

- Loneliness rates have been increasing since the 1970s.
- Social isolation increases mortality risk by 26 to 29 percent.
- Quality conversations boost well-being.
- Community engagement enhances growth.

PRACTICAL ACTIONS

1. ASSESS YOUR PASSION BALANCE

- Complete the passion scale assessment.
- Calculate harmonious versus obsessive scores.
- Identify areas of imbalance.
- Work toward more harmonious engagement.

2. DESIGN YOUR ENVIRONMENT

- Create systems that reduce reliance on willpower.
- Set up your space to support desired behaviors.
- Remove unnecessary friction points.
- Make good choices more automatic.

3. BUILD MEANINGFUL CONNECTIONS

- Set aside dedicated connection time.
- Focus on quality over quantity.
- Engage in authentic self-expression.
- Consider community involvement.

Remember This

True self-improvement isn't self-centered—it's self-expanding. Sustainable growth comes from balancing personal development with meaningful connections and contributions to others.

Looking Ahead

As we conclude, consider how you can apply these principles to create your regenerative approach to performance and well-being.

EPILOGUE

After two decades immersed in human performance science, I've witnessed something paradoxical: As our knowledge of optimization has expanded, our sense of well-being has contracted. We wake up earlier, track more, and optimize harder—yet satisfaction remains elusive. The self-improvement industry grows relentlessly, while mental health statistics move in the opposite direction.

This book began by questioning why our sophisticated approaches to performance often leave us feeling more depleted than empowered. We've explored why elaborate morning routines have become modern secular rituals, why time seems to slip through our fingers despite productivity apps and life hacks, and why sleep remains mysterious despite wearable technologies that track our every toss and turn. We've examined the puzzling reality that despite record gym membership numbers, overall fitness levels are declining and why nutrition science seems to contradict itself with each passing month.

Most crucially, we've confronted the central paradox of modern work: As physical labor decreases, mental exhaustion soars. Our bodies sit in ergonomic chairs while our minds run ultramarathons.

The answers we've uncovered point to a fundamental truth: Human performance isn't a code to be cracked but a garden to be tended. The path forward lies neither in the seductive promises of *hyperoptimizers* nor in the resigned withdrawal of *quiet quitters*. It exists neither in the burnout-bound lanes of *hustle culture* nor in the unfulfilled comfort of the *soft life*.

Instead, *Regenerative Performance* offers a middle path—one that honors both ambition and sustainability, excellence and recovery, growth and grace. This approach recognizes that peak performance isn't about perpetual maximization but rather about the rhythmic oscillation between challenge and renewal.

As you close this book, you now possess tools that transcend simple optimization. You understand why working harder isn't always working better, why rest is a skill as crucial as effort, and why sustainable success requires periods of strategic renewal. Most importantly, you recognize that true performance isn't a solo journey but one enriched by connection and community.

The challenges of our *always-on* world won't disappear tomorrow. The pressure to optimize every aspect of existence won't evaporate. But you now have a framework for navigating these waters with greater wisdom and resilience. You can pursue excellence without sacrificing well-being, push boundaries without breaking yourself, and achieve meaningful goals while maintaining vital connections.

This is the essence of *Regenerative Performance*—not a finish line to cross but a way of moving through the world. It's about building capacity rather than just spending it, growing stronger through challenges rather than being diminished by it, and finding flow in the rhythm of effort and renewal.

The journey ahead is yours to shape. May you walk it with confidence, clarity, and the knowledge that sustainable success isn't about perpetual optimization—it's about intentional regeneration.

Welcome to your next chapter.

Explore Further Resources

Your journey toward *Regenerative Performance* doesn't end here. To help you implement the concepts and strategies outlined in this book, I've created a collection of tools and resources that you can access on my website.

drjameshewitt.com/regenerativeperformance

Stay Connected

I'd love to hear how *Regenerative Performance* has influenced you. Share your story or connect with me directly by signing up for my newsletter or following me on social media.

Newsletter: Stay updated with new articles, insights, and tools.

Social Media: Follow me on LinkedIn or Instagram for regular tips and inspiration.

ENDNOTES

1   B. Franklin, *Poor Richard's Almanack: Selections from the Apothegms and Proverbs* (London: Forgotten Books, 2018).

2   D. A. Kalmbach et al., "Genetic Basis of Chronotype in Humans: Insights from Three Landmark GWAS," *Sleep* 40 (2017).

3   D. Fischer et al., "Chronotypes in the US—Influence of Age and Sex," *PLoS One* 12 no. 6 (June 21, 2017).

4   Alexander A. Borbély et al, "The two-process model of sleep regulation: a reappraisal," *Journal of Sleep Research* 25, no. 2 (2016): 131–43.

5   H. P. Landolt, "Sleep Homeostasis: A Role for Adenosine in Humans?" *Biochem Pharmacol* 75, no. 11 (June 1, 2008): 2070–9.

6   J. F. Duffy, D. W. Rimmer, and C. A. Czeisler, "Association of Intrinsic Circadian Period with Morningness-Eveningness, Usual Wake Time, and Circadian Phase," *Behavioral Neuroscience* 115 no. 4 (2001): 895–9.

7   D. J. Dijk and S. W. Lockley, "Integration of human sleep-wake regulation and circadian rhythmicity," *Journal of Applied Physiology* 92, no. 2 (2002): 852–62.

8   S. W. Lockley et al., "Alertness, mood and performance rhythm disturbances associated with circadian sleep disorders in the blind," *Journal of Sleep Research* 17, no. 2 (2008): 207–16.

9   M. Stolarski and J. Gorgol, "Analyzing Social Perception of Chronotypes Within the Stereotype Content Model," *Chronobiol Int* 39, no. 11 (2022): 1475–84.

10 K. C. Yam, R. Fehr, and C. M. Barnes, "Morning Employees Are Perceived as Better Employees: Employees' Start Times Influence Supervisor Performance Ratings," *Journal of Applied Psychology* 99, no. 6 (Nov. 1, 2014): 1288–99.

11 Z. Owen et al., "Lingering Impacts on Sleep Following the Daylight Savings Time Transition in the Project Baseline Health Study," *Sleep Sci Pract* [Internet] 6, no. 1 (2022): 13.

12 C. von Gall et al., "Chronotype-Dependent Sleep Loss Is Associated with a Lower Amplitude in Circadian Rhythm and a Higher Fragmentation of REM Sleep in Young Healthy Adults," *Brain Sci* 13, no. 10 (Oct. 19, 2023).

13 J. Costa-Font, S. Fleche, and R. Pagan, "The Welfare Effects of Time Reallocation: Evidence from Daylight Saving Time," *Economica* 91, no. 362 (Apr. 1, 2024): 547–68.

14 S. Tanaka and H. Koizumi, "Springing Forward and Falling Back on Health: The Effect of Daylight Saving Time on Acute Myocardial Infarction," *medRxiv preprint* [Internet] (2022): 1–69.

15 B. Kolla et al., "0173 Spring Forward, Fall Back: Increased Patient Safety-Related Adverse Events Following the Spring Time Change," *Sleep* 43 (2020): A69.

16 A. C. Smith, "Spring Forward at Your Own Risk: Daylight Saving Time and Fatal Vehicle Crashes," *Am Econ J Appl Econ* 8, no. 2 (2016): 65–91.

17 S. Leahy et al., "Associations between Circadian Alignment and Cognitive Functioning in a Nationally Representative Sample of Older Adults," *Sci Rep* 14, no. 1 (June 12, 2024).

18 K. M. Bermingham et al., "Exploring the Relationship between Social Jetlag with Gut Microbial Composition, Diet and Cardiometabolic Health, in the ZOE PREDICT 1 Cohort," *Eur J Nutr* 62, no. 8 (Dec. 1, 2023): 3135–47.

19 G. L. Ottoni, E. Antoniolli, and D. R. Lara, "The Circadian Energy Scale (CIRENS): Two Simple Questions for a Reliable Chronotype Measurement Based on Energy," *Chronobiol Int* 28, no. 3 (April 2011): 229–37.

20 D. Kocevska et al., "Heritability of Sleep Duration and Quality: A Systematic Review and Meta-Analysis," *Sleep Med Rev* 59 (Oct. 1, 2021).

21 M. A. Bonmati-Carrion et al., "Protecting the Melatonin Rhythm through Circadian Healthy Light Exposure," *Int J Mol Sci* 15, no. 12 (2014): 23448–500.

22 S. L. Chellappa, C. J. Morris, and F. A. J. L. Scheer, "Daily Circadian Misalignment Impairs Human Cognitive Performance Task-Dependently," *Sci Rep* 8, no. 1 (2018): 1–11.

23 S. M. Mattingly et al., "Snoozing: An Examination of a Common Method of Waking," *Sleep* 45, no. 10 (Oct. 1, 2022).

24 M. Arain et al., "Maturation of the Adolescent Brain," *Neuropsychiatr Dis Treat* 9 (2013): 449–61.

25 T. Sundelin, S. Landry, and J. Axelsson, "Is Snoozing Losing? Why Intermittent Morning Alarms Are Used and How They Affect Sleep, Cognition, Cortisol, and Mood," *J Sleep Res* 33, no. 3 (May 1, 2024).

26 T. L. Sletten et al., "The Importance of Sleep Regularity: A Consensus Statement of the National Sleep Foundation Sleep Timing and Variability Panel," *Sleep Health* 9, no. 6 (Dec. 1, 2023): 801–20.

27 G. Loewenstein, "Self-Control and Its Discontents: A Commentary on Duckworth, Milkman, and Laibson," *Psychological Science in the Public Interest* 19, no. 3 (Dec. 1, 2018): 95–101.

28 J. Colin et al., "Rhythm of the Rectal Temperature during a Six-Month Free-Running Experiment," *J Appl Physiol* 25, no. 1 (1968): 170–6.

29 T. M. Brown et al., "Recommendations for Daytime, Evening, and Nighttime Indoor Light Exposure to Best Support Physiology, Sleep, and Wakefulness in Healthy Adults," *PLoS Biol* 20, no. 3 (Mar. 17, 2022).

30 C. Blume, C. Garbazza, and M. Spitschan, "Effects of light on human circadian rhythms, sleep and mood." *Somnologie : Schlafforschung und Schlafmedizin = Somnology : sleep research and sleep medicine* 23, no. 3 (2019): 147–56.

31 A. D. M. Koopman et al., "The Association between Social Jetlag, the Metabolic Syndrome, and Type 2 Diabetes Mellitus in the General Population: The New Hoorn Study," *Journal of Biological Rhythms* 32, no. 4 (2017): 359–68.

32 J. Antonio et al., "Common Questions and Misconceptions about Caffeine Supplementation: What Does the Scientific Evidence Really Show?" *Journal of the International Society of Sports Nutrition* 21 (2024).

33 A. Nehlig, J. L. Daval, and G. Debry, "Caffeine and the Central Nervous System: Mechanisms of Action, Biochemical, Metabolic and Psychostimulant Effects," *Brain Res* 17, no. 2 (1992): 139–70.

34 E. Murillo-Rodriguez et al., "The Diurnal Rhythm of Adenosine Levels in the Basal Forebrain of Young and Old Rats," *Neuroscience* 123, no. 2 (2004): 361–70.

35 C. F. Reichert, T. Deboer, and H. P. Landolt, "Adenosine, Caffeine, and Sleep–Wake Regulation: State of the Science and Perspectives," *Journal of Sleep Research* 31 (2022).

36 T. Porkka-Heiskanen et al., "Adenosine: A Mediator of the Sleep-Inducing Effects of Prolonged Wakefulness," *Science* 276 (1997).

37 N. Rieth et al., "Caffeine and Saliva Steroids in Young Healthy Recreationally Trained Women: Impact of Regular Caffeine Intake," *Endocrine* 52 (2016): 391–4.

38 J. Grgic et al., "Wake Up and Smell the Coffee: Caffeine Supplementation and Exercise Performance—An Umbrella Review of 21 Published Meta-Analyses," *Br J Sports Med* 54, no. 11 (June 1, 2020).

39 D. Chieng et al., "The Impact of Coffee Subtypes on Incident Cardiovascular Disease, Arrhythmias, and Mortality: Long-Term Outcomes from the UK Biobank," *Eur J Prev Cardiol* 29, no. 17 (Dec. 7, 2022): 2240–9.

40 R. Poole et al., "Coffee Consumption and Health: Umbrella Review of Meta-Analyses of Multiple Health Outcomes," *BMJ* 359 (Nov. 22, 2017): j5024.

41 Grand View Research, "Global Cold Plunge Tub Market Size & Outlook, 2023–2030" (2023).

42 Y. Ravussin et al., "Effect of Intermittent Cold Exposure on Brown Fat Activation, Obesity, and Energy Homeostasis in Mice," *PLoS One* 9, no. 1 (Jan. 17, 2014).

43 S. Mondal et al., "MiRNA and Leptin Signaling in Metabolic Diseases and at Extreme Environments," *Pharmacology Research and Perspectives* 12 (2024).

44 S. Pani et al., "Brown to White Fat Transition Overlap with Skeletal Muscle during Development of Larger Mammals: Is It a Coincidence?" *Journal of the Endocrine Society* 6 (2022).

45 C. J. Gordon, "Thermal Physiology of Laboratory Mice: Defining Thermoneutrality," *Journal of Thermal Biology* 37 (2012): 654–85.

46 Retraction: J. Néma et al., "Impact of cold exposure on life satisfaction and physical composition of soldiers," *BMJ Military Health* 170 (Jan. 29, 2024).

47 C. Benedict et al., "Acute Sleep Deprivation Enhances the Brain's Response to Hedonic Food Stimuli: An fMRI Study," *Journal of Clinical Endocrinology and Metabolism* 97, no. 3 (March 2012).

48 J. P. Thyfault and A. Bergouignan, "Exercise and Metabolic Health: Beyond Skeletal Muscle," *Diabetologia* 63, no. 8 (Aug. 1, 2020): 1464–74.

49 D. S. Weisberg et al., "The Seductive Allure of Neuroscience Explanations," *J Cogn Neurosci* 20, no. 3 (Mar. 1, 2008): 470–7.

50 P. Srámek et al., "Human Physiological Responses to Immersion into Water of Different Temperatures," *Eur J Appl Physiol* 81, no. 5 (2000): 436–42.

51 R. C. Sellnow et al., "Regulation of dopamine neurotransmission from serotonergic neurons by ectopic expression of the dopamine D2 autoreceptor blocks levodopa-induced dyskinesia," *Acta Neuropathologica Communications*, 7, no. 1 (2019): 8.

52 M. Falla et al., "The Effect of Cold Exposure on Cognitive Performance in Healthy Adults: A Systematic Review," *International Journal of Environmental Research and Public Health* 18 (2021).

53 G. D. Stanwood, "Dopamine and Stress," in *Stress: Physiology, Biochemistry, and Pathology*, ed. G. Fink (London: Academic Press, 2019), 105–14.

54 J. C. Basso and W. A. Suzuki, "The Effects of Acute Exercise on Mood, Cognition, Neurophysiology, and Neurochemical Pathways: A Review," *Brain Plast* 2 (2017): 127–52.

55 J. Reed and D. S. Ones, "The Effect of Acute Aerobic Exercise on Positive Activated Affect: A Meta-Analysis," *Psychol Sport Exerc* 7, no. 5 (2006): 477–514.

56 M. J. Tipton et al., "Cold Water Immersion: Kill or Cure?" *Exp Physiol* 102, no. 11 (Nov. 1, 2017): 1335–55.

57 M. J. Shattock and M. J. Tipton, "'Autonomic Conflict': A Different Way to Die during Cold Water Immersion?" *Journal of Physiology* 590 (2012): 3219–30.

58 D. J. Clayton and L. J. James, "The Effect of Breakfast on Appetite Regulation, Energy Balance and Exercise Performance," *Proceedings of the Nutrition Society* 75, no. 3 (2016): 319–27.

59 C. L. Yang and R. M. Tucker, "Beneficial Effects of a High Protein Breakfast on Fullness Disappear after a Night of Short Sleep in Nonobese, Premenopausal Women," *Physiol Behav* 229 (Feb. 1, 2021).

60 E. J. Dhurandhar et al., "The Effectiveness of Breakfast Recommendations on Weight Loss: A Randomized Controlled Trial," *American Journal of Clinical Nutrition* 100, no. 2 (2014): 507–13.

61 L. B. Dalgaard et al., "A Dairy-Based, Protein-Rich Breakfast Enhances Satiety and Cognitive Concentration before Lunch in Overweight to Obese Young Females: A Randomized Controlled Crossover Study," *J Dairy Sci* 107, no. 5 (May 1, 2024): 2653–67.

62 J. Fulford, J. L. Varley-Campbell, and C. A. Williams, "The Effect of Breakfast versus No Breakfast on Brain Activity in Adolescents When Performing Cognitive Tasks, as Assessed by fMRI," *Nutr Neurosci* 19, no. 3 (2016): 110–5.

63 I. Iovino et al., "Breakfast Consumption Has No Effect on Neuropsychological Functioning in Children: A Repeated-Measures Clinical Trial," *American Journal of Clinical Nutrition* 104, no. 3 (Sep. 1, 2016): 715–21.

64 N. Giménez-Legarre et al., "Breakfast Characteristics and Its Association with Daily Micronutrients Intake in Children and Adolescents—A Systematic Review and Meta-Analysis," *Nutrients* 12 (2020): 1–23.

65 M. Nashrudin Bin Naharudin et al., "Breakfast Omission Reduces Subsequent Resistance Exercise Performance," *J Strength Cond Res* [Internet] 33, no. 7 (2019): 1766–72. Available from www.nsca.com.

66 S. A. Mears et al., "Perception of Breakfast Ingestion Enhances High-Intensity Cycling Performance," *Int J Sports Physiol Perform* 13, no. 4 (Apr. 1, 2018): 504–9.

67 Microsoft, *2022 Work Trend Index: Annual Report* (2022).

68 S. G. Rogelberg, *The Cost of Unnecessary Meeting Attendance* (2022).

69 D. Smith, "50 Surprising Meeting Statistics for 2024," *Flowtrace* (2024).

70 Qatalog and GitLab, "Killing Time at Work '22" (2022).

71 Slack Workforce Lab, "The Data-Driven Secret to a Productive Work Day" (2023).

72 G. Mark, G. Daniela, and U. Klocke, "The Cost of Interrupted Work: More Speed and Stress," CHI '08: Proceedings of the SIGCHI Conference on Human Factors in Computing Systems [Internet] (2008), 107–10.

73 Microsoft, "Will AI Fix Work? 2023 Work Trend Index" (2023).

74 T. W. Jackson, R. Dawson, and D. Wilson, "Understanding Email Interaction Increases Organizational Productivity," *Commun ACM* 46, no. 8 (2003): 80–4.

75 QS Supplies, "Tweeting on the Toilet," 2021.

76 Economist Impact, "In Search of Lost Focus: Productivity in the Post-Pandemic World" [Internet] (2023).

77 Gartner, "Gartner HR Research Identifies New Framework for Organizations to Succeed in Today's Fragmented Workplace" (2022).

78 O. Bouwmeester et al., "Accentuating Dirty Work: Coping with Psychological Taint in Elite Management Consulting," *German Journal of Human Resource Management: Zeitschrift für Personalforschung* 239700222110554 (2021).

79   J. Hewitt, *Wellbeing and Performance in Always-On Knowledge Work: A Multifaceted Investigation Using Digital Phenotyping* (Loughborough University, 2023).

80   J. Harter, "Is Quiet Quitting Real?" vol. 6 (2022), https://www.gallup.com/workplace/398306/quiet-quitting-real.aspx.

81   T. Mahand and C. Caldwell, "Quiet Quitting—Causes and Opportunities," *Business and Management Research* 12, no. 1 (Jan. 9, 2023): 9–19.

82   E. Tønnessen et al., "The Road to Gold: Training and Peaking Characteristics in the Year Prior to a Gold Medal Endurance Performance," *PLoS One* 9, no. 7 (July 14, 2014).

83   T. Stöggl and B. Sperlich, "Polarized Training Has Greater Impact on Key Endurance Variables than Threshold, High Intensity, or High Volume Training," *Front Physiol* (Feb. 4, 2014).

84   J. Hewitt, "Human Intelligence," in *Exponential*, eds. J. Hewitt and A. Hintsa (Helsinki, Finland: Hintsa Performance, 2016), 80–105.

85   G. Wainstein et al., "The Role of the Locus Coeruleus in Shaping Adaptive Cortical Melodies," *Trends in Cognitive Sciences* 26 (2022): 527–38.

86   M. Storoni, *Hyperefficient: Simple Methods to Optimise Your Brain and Transform the Way You Work* (London: Yellow Kite, 2024).

87   D. Robson, "Take Control of Your Brain's Master Switch to Optimise How You Think," *New Scientist* (2024).

88   H. Cao et al., "Large Scale Analysis of Multitasking Behavior during Remote Meetings," in *Conference on Human Factors in Computing Systems—Proceedings* (Association for Computing Machinery, 2021).

89   M. Arena, "Beware of the Activity Avalanche That Can Damage Employee Well-Being," *HR Exchange Network* (2023).

90   Worklytics, "Activity Avalanche: How Return-to-Office Is Impacting Collaboration" (2022).

91   R. Hougaard and J. Carter, "If You Aspire to Be a Great Leader, Be Present," in *Mindful Listening* (HBR emotional intelligence series), eds. J. Zenger, J. Carter, P. Bregman, and R. Hougaard (Harvard Business Press, 2019).

92   B. Laker et al., "Dear Manager, You're Holding Too Many Meetings," *Harvard Business Review* (Mar. 9, 2022).

93   E. Russell et al., "Getting on Top of Work-Email: A Systematic Review of 25 Years of Research to Understand Effective Work-Email Activity," *J Occup Organ Psychol* 97, no. 1 (Mar. 1, 2024): 74–103.

94   G. Mark, M. Czerwinski, and S. T. Iqbal, "Effects of Individual Differences in Blocking Workplace Distractions," in *Conference on Human Factors in Computing Systems—Proceedings* (Association for Computing Machinery, 2018).

95   G. Mark et al., "Email Duration, Batching and Self-Interruption: Patterns of Email Use on Productivity and Stress," in *CHI '16: Proceedings of the 2016 CHI Conference on Human Factors in Computing Systems* (Association for Computing Machinery, 2016), 1717–28.

96   C. Callahan, "How Asana and Slack's Meeting Purges Have Paid Off," *WorkLife.news* (2024).

97   C. B. Hines, "Time-of-Day Effects on Human Performance," *Catholic Education: A Journal of Inquiry and Practice* 7, no. 3 (2004): 390–413.

98   S. W. Lockley and R. G. Foster, *Sleep: A Very Short Introduction* (Oxford: Oxford University Press, 2012).

99   A. F. Ward et al., "Brain Drain: The Mere Presence of One's Own Smartphone Reduces Available Cognitive Capacity," *J Assoc Consum Res* 2, no. 2 (Apr. 1, 2017): 140–54.

100   J. T. Dean, "Noise, Cognitive Function, and Worker Productivity," *Am Econ J Appl Econ* 16, no. 4 (2024): 322–60.

101   S. Romano et al., "The Effect of Noise on Software Engineers' Performance," in *Proceedings of ACM Conference, Washington, DC, USA, July 2017* (Conference '17, 2018), 1–10.

102   C. Cajochen et al., "Dose-Response Relationship for Light Intensity and Ocular and Electroencephalographic Correlates of Human Alertness" [Internet] *Behavioural Brain Research* 115 (2000).

103   R. Golmohammadi et al., "Effects of Light on Attention and Reaction Time: A Systematic Review," *J Res Health Sci* 21, no. 4 (Oct. 31, 2021).

104   J. M. Watson and D. L. Strayer, "Supertaskers: Profiles in Extraordinary Multitasking Ability," *Psychon Bull Rev* 17, no. 4 (2010): 479–85.

105   S. Conte, F. Ferlazzo, and P. Renzi, "Ultradian Rhythms of Reaction Times in Performance in Vigilance Tasks," *Biol Psychol* 39, nos. 2–3 (1995): 159–72.

106   C. Nakatani, B. Ganschow, and C. van Leeuwen, "Long-Term Dynamics of Mind Wandering: Ultradian Rhythms in Thought Generation," *Neurosci Conscious* 2019, no. 1 (2019): 1–12.

107 Microsoft, "Research Proves Your Brain Needs Breaks" (April 2021).

108 P. Albulescu et al., "'Give Me a Break!' A Systematic Review and Meta-Analysis on the Efficacy of Micro-Breaks for Increasing Well-Being and Performance," *PLoS One* 17 (2022).

109 S. Kim, Y. A. Park, and L. Headrick, "Daily Micro-Breaks and Job Performance: General Work Engagement as a Cross-Level Moderator," *Journal of Applied Psychology* 103, no. 7 (2018): 772–86.

110 A. J. Oswald, E. Proto, and D. Sgroi, "Happiness and Productivity," *J Labor Econ* 33 no. 4 (2015): 789–821, http://webarchive.national.

111 M. Luo, A. Falisi, and J. Hancock, "Can Text Messaging Influence Perceptions of Geographical Slant? A Replication and Extension of Schnall, Harber, Stefanucci, and Proffitt (2008)." *Technology, Mind, and Behavior* 2, no. 2 (2021).

112 K. M. Diaz et al., "Patterns of Sedentary Behavior and Mortality in U.S. Middle-Aged and Older Adults: A National Cohort Study," *Ann Intern Med* 167, no. 7 (2017): 465–75.

113 M. Oppezzo and D. L. Schwartz, "Give Your Ideas Some Legs: The Positive Effect of Walking on Creative Thinking," *J Exp Psychol Learn Mem Cogn* 40, no. 4 (2014): 1142–52.

114 S. Kaplan, "The Restorative Benefits of Nature: Toward an Integrative Framework," *J Environ Psychol* 15, no. 3 (1995): 169–82.

115 M. G. Berman, J. Jonides, and S. Kaplan, "The Cognitive Benefits of Interacting with Nature," *Psychol Sci* 19, no. 12 (2008): 1207–12, http://www.sacklerinstitute.org/.

116 C. M. Hagerhall et al., "Investigations of Human EEG Response to Viewing Fractal Patterns," *Perception* 37, no. 10 (2008): 1488–94.

117 C. Song, H. Ikei, and Y. Miyazaki, "Effects of Forest-Derived Visual, Auditory, and Combined Stimuli," *Urban For Urban Green* 64 (Sep. 1, 2021).

118 H. Jo, C. Song, and Y. Miyazaki, "Physiological Benefits of Viewing Nature: A Systematic Review of Indoor Experiments," *International Journal of Environmental Research and Public Health* 16 (2019).

119 N. C. Andreasen, "A Journey into Chaos: Creativity and the Unconscious," *Mens Sana Monograpas* 9 (2011): 42–53.

120 WFHResearch, "Survey of Working Arrangement and Attitudes: July 2023," (July 2023).

121 A. E. Reinberg et al., "Seven-Day Human Biological Rhythms: An Expedition in Search of Their Origin, Synchronization, Functional Advantage, Adaptive Value and Clinical Relevance," *Chronobiol Int* 34, no. 2 (Feb. 7, 2017): 162–91.

122 F. Levi and F. Halberg, "Circaseptan (about-7-Day) Bioperiodicity—Spontaneous and Reactive—and the Search for Pacemakers," *Ricerca in Clinica e in Laboratorio* 12, no. 2 (1982): 323.

123 S. Sonnentag and C. Fritz, "The Recovery Experience Questionnaire: Development and Validation of a Measure for Assessing Recuperation and Unwinding from Work," *J Occup Health Psychol* 12, no. 3 (2007) 204–21.

124 Business in the Community. "Your job can be good for you: Backing business to revolutionise ways of working in the UK," BITC Wellbeing Leadership Team (2022).

125 D. Gallie, M. White, and Y. Cheng, *Restructuring the Employment Relationship* (Oxford: Clarendon Press, 1998).

126 D. Gallie and M. White, "Employment in Britain Survey" (1992).

127 N. Singer-Velush, "Why Unplugging from Work Is More Work than We Think," *Microsoft Workplace Insights* (2019).

128 L. H. L. Liang, "The Psychology behind 'Revenge Bedtime Procrastination,'" British Broadcasting Corporation (2020), https://www.bbc.com/worklife/article/20201123-the-psychology-behind-revenge-bedtime-procrastination.

129 J. Pietilä et al., "Acute Effect of Alcohol Intake on Cardiovascular Autonomic Regulation during the First Hours of Sleep in a Large Real-World Sample of Finnish Employees: Observational Study," *JMIR Ment Health* 5, no. 1 (2018): 1–13.

130 S. Sonnentag, "The Recovery Paradox: Portraying the Complex Interplay between Job Stressors, Lack of Recovery, and Poor Well-Being," *Res Organ Behav* 38 (2018): 169–85, https://doi.org/10.1016/j.riob.2018.11.002.

131 G. E. Kreiner, "Consequences of Work-Home Segmentation or Integration: A Person-Environment Fit Perspective," *J Organ Behav* 27, no. 4 (2006): 485–507.

132 A. Firoozabadi, S. Uitdewilligen, and F. R. H. Zijlstra, "Solving Problems or Seeing Troubles? A Day-Level Study on the Consequences of Thinking about Work on Recovery and Well-Being, and the Moderating Role of Self-Regulation," *European Journal of Work and Organizational Psychology* 27, no. 5 (2018): 629–41.

133 M. Cropley and F. R. H. Zijlstra, "Work and rumination," in *Handbook of Stress in the Occupations*, eds. C. Cooper and J. Langan-Fox (Cheltenham: Edward Elgar, 2011), 487–503.

134 J. Becker and J. Lanzl, "Segmentation Preference and Technostress: Integrators' vs Segmenters' Experience of Technology-Induced Demands and Related Spill-Over Effects," *Information and Management* 60, no. 5 (July 1, 2023).

135 D. S. Carlson et al., "Boundary Management Tactics: Aligning Preferences in the Work and Family Domains," *Academy of Management Proceedings* 2013, no. 1 (2013): 11061.

136 R. Fuller, N. Shikaloff, R. Cullinan, and S. Harmon, "If you multitask during meetings, your team will, too," *Harvard Business Review*, January 25, 2018.

137 M. Cropley and L. J. Millward, "How Do Individuals 'Switch-Off' from Work during Leisure? A Qualitative Description of the Unwinding Process in High and Low Ruminators," *Leisure Studies* 28, no. 3 (2009): 333–47.

138 D. Etzion, D. Eden, and Y. Lapidot, "Relief from Job Stressors and Burnout: Reserve Service as a Respite" (September 1998).

139 T. Åkerstedt et al., "Sleep Disturbances, Work Stress and Work Hours: A Cross-Sectional Study," *J Psychosom Res* 53, no. 3 (2002): 741–8.

140 M. Cropley, D. J. Dijk, and N. Stanley, "Job Strain, Work Rumination, and Sleep in School Teachers," *European Journal of Work and Organizational Psychology* 15, no. 2 (2006): 181–96.

141 L. Nylén, B. Melin, and L. Laflamme, "Interference between Work and Outside-Work Demands Relative to Health: Unwinding Possibilities among Full-Time and Part-Time Employees," *International Journal of Behavioral Medicine* 14 (2007).

142 G. Pravettoni et al., "The Differential Role of Mental Rumination among Industrial and Knowledge Workers," *Ergonomics* 50, no. 11 (November 2007): 1931–40.

143 P. Suadicani, H. O. Hein, and F. Gyntelberg, "Are Social Inequalities as Associated with the Risk of Ischaemic Heart Disease a Result of Psychosocial Working Conditions?" *Atherosclerosis* 101, no. 2 (1993): 165–75.

144 B. S. McEwen, "Stress, Adaptation, and Disease. Allostasis and Allostatic Load," *Ann NY Acad Sci* 840 (May 1, 1998): 33–44.

145 A. Firoozabadi, S. Uitdewilligen, and F. R. H. Zijlstra, "Should You Switch Off or Stay Engaged? The Consequences of Thinking about Work on the Trajectory of Psychological Well-Being Over Time," *J Occup Health Psychol* 23, no. 2 (2018): 278–88.

146 S. Sonnentag and U. V. Bayer, "Switching off Mentally: Predictors and Consequences of Psychological Detachment from Work during Off-Job Time," *J Occup Health Psychol* 10, no. 4 (2005): 393–414.

147 K. Perko, U. Kinnunen, and T. Feldt, "Long-Term Profiles of Work-Related Rumination Associated with Leadership, Job Demands, and Exhaustion: A Three-Wave Study," *Work Stress* 31, no. 4 (2017): 395–420.

148 B. Zeigarnik, "Das Behalten erledigter und unerledigter Handlungen," *Psychol Forsch* 9 (1938): 1–85.

149 R. M. Ryan, J. G. LaGuardia, and L. J. Rawsthorne, "Self-Complexity and the Authenticity of Self-Aspects: Effects on Well Being and Resilience to Stressful Events," *N Am J Psychol* 7, no. 3 (2005): 431–48.

150 R. Raphael, "Netflix CEO Reed Hastings: Sleep Is Our Competition," *Fast Company* (2017).

151 S. Battams et al., "Workplace Risk Factors for Anxiety and Depression in Male-Dominated Industries: A Systematic Review," *Health Psychol Behav Med* 2, no. 1 (2014): 983–1008.

152 A. M. Roche et al., "Alcohol Use among Workers in Male-Dominated Industries: A Systematic Review of Risk Factors," *Saf Sci* 78 (2015): 124–41.

153 M. Virtanen et al., "Long Working Hours and Alcohol Use: Systematic Review and Meta-Analysis of Published Studies and Unpublished Individual Participant Data," *BMJ* [Internet] 350 (January 2015): 1–14.

154 E. Goddard, *Smoking and Drinking among Adults, 2006* (2006).

155 M. L. Cooper et al., "Drinking to Regulate Positive and Negative Emotions: A Motivational Model of Alcohol Use," *J Pers Soc Psychol* 69, no. 5 (1995): 990–1005.

156 R. A. Hendler et al., "Stimulant and Sedative Effects of Alcohol," *Behavioral Neurobiology of Alcohol Addiction* 13 (2013): 489–509.

157 J. Studer et al., "Drinking Motives as Mediators of the Associations between Reinforcement Sensitivity and Alcohol Misuse and Problems," *Front Psychol* 7 (May 2016): 1–12.

158 M. E. Patrick, C. M. Lee, and M. E. Larimer, "Drinking Motives, Protective Behavioral Strategies, and Experienced Consequences: Identifying Students at Risk," *Addictive Behaviour* 36, no. 3 (2011): 270–3.

159 G. N. Pires et al., "Effects of Acute Sleep Deprivation on State Anxiety Levels: A Systematic Review and Meta-Analysis," *Sleep Med* [Internet] 24 (2016): 109–18.

160 E. Gonzalez-Mulé and B. S. Cockburn, "This Job Is (Literally) Killing Me: A Moderated-Mediated Model Linking Work Characteristics to Mortality," *Journal of Applied Psychology* 106 (2020).

161 Edelman, *Edelman Trust Barometer* (2023).

162 C. Fritz and S. Sonnentag, "Recovery, Well-Being, and Performance-Related Outcomes: The Role of Workload and Vacation Experiences," *Journal of Applied Psychology* 91, no. 4 (July 2006): 936–45.

163 E. J. Masicampo and R. F. Baumeister, "Consider It Done! Plan Making Can Eliminate the Cognitive Effects of Unfulfilled Goals," *J Pers Soc Psychol* 101, no. 4 (2011): 667–83.

164 J. Wendsche and A. Lohmann-Haislah, "A Meta-Analysis on Antecedents and Outcomes of Detachment from Work," *Front Psychol* 7 (January 2017): 1–24.

165 K. Lanaj, A. S. Gabriel, and R. E. Jennings, "The Importance of Leader Recovery for Leader Identity and Behavior," *Journal of Applied Psychology* 108, no. 10 (Apr. 6, 2023): 1717–36.

166 T. J. S. Koch et al., "Psychological Detachment Matters Right after Work: Engaging in Physical Exercise after Stressful Workdays," *Int J Stress Manag* 31 (July 18, 2024).

167 C. R. Patterson, J. B. Bennett, and W. L. Wiitala, "Healthy and Unhealthy Stress Unwinding: Promoting Health in Small Businesses," *J Bus Psychol* 20, no. 2 (2005): 221–47.

168 N. Feuerhahn, S. Sonnentag, and A. Woll, "Exercise after Work, Psychological Mediators, and Affect: A Day-Level Study," *European Journal of Work and Organizational Psychology* 23, no. 1 (2014): 62–79.

169 S. Sonnentag, "Work, Recovery Activities, and Individual Well-Being: A Diary Study," *J Occup Health Psychol* 6, no. 3 (2001): 196–210.

170 T. Karabinski et al., "Interventions for Improving Psychological Detachment from Work: A Meta-Analysis," *J Occup Health Psychol* 26, no. 3 (2021): 224–42.

171 A. Gawor, E. Hogervorst, and T. Wilcockson, "Does an Acute Bout of Moderate Exercise Reduce Alcohol Craving in University Students?" *Addictive Behaviors* 123, no. 107071 (2021).

172 P. H. P. Hanel et al., "Value Fulfillment and Well-Being: Clarifying Directions Over Time," *J Pers* 92, no. 4 (Aug. 1, 2024): 1037–49.

173 A. Bolwerk et al., "How Art Changes Your Brain: Differential Effects of Visual Art Production and Cognitive Art Evaluation on Functional Brain Connectivity," *PLoS One* 9, no. 7 (July 1, 2014).

174 T. M. Brown et al., "Recommendations for Daytime, Evening, and Nighttime Indoor Light Exposure to Best Support Physiology, Sleep, and Wakefulness in Healthy Adults," *PLoS Biol* 20, no. 3 (Mar. 1, 2022).

175 Y. Ooishi et al., "Increase in Salivary Oxytocin and Decrease in Salivary Cortisol after Listening to Relaxing Slow-Tempo and Exciting Fast-Tempo Music," *PLoS One* 12, no. 12 (Dec. 1, 2017).

176 P. R. Steffen et al., "The Impact of Resonance Frequency Breathing on Measures of Heart Rate Variability, Blood Pressure, and Mood," *Front Public Health* 5 (August 2017): 6–11.

177 A. Zaccaro et al., "How Breath-Control Can Change Your Life: A Systematic Review on Psycho-Physiological Correlates of Slow Breathing," *Front Hum Neurosci* 12 (September 2018): 1–16.

178 J. A. Waxenbaum, V. Reddy, and M. Varacallo, *Anatomy, Autonomic Nervous System* (Treasure Island, Florida: StatPearls [Internet], 2022).

179 Q. Chang, R. Liu, and Z. Shen, "Effects of Slow Breathing Rate on Blood Pressure and Heart Rate Variabilities," *Int J Cardiol* 169, no. 1 (Oct. 25, 2013).

180 P. Z. Zhang et al., "Respiration Response Curve Analysis of Heart Rate Variability," *IEEE Trans Biomed Eng* 44, no. 4 (1997): 321.

181 G. K. Pal, S. Velkumary, and Madanmohan, "Effect of Short-Term Practice of Breathing Exercises on Autonomic Functions in Normal Human Volunteers," *Indian J Med Res* 120, no. 2 (2004): 115–21.

182 X. Yu et al., "Activation of the Anterior Prefrontal Cortex and Serotonergic System Is Associated with Improvements in Mood and EEG Changes Induced by Zen Meditation Practice in Novices," *International Journal of Psychophysiology* 80, no. 2 (May 2011): 103–11.

183 M. Fumoto et al., "Appearance of High-Frequency Alpha Band with Disappearance of Low-Frequency Alpha Band in EEG Is Produced during Voluntary Abdominal Breathing in an Eyes-Closed Condition," *Neurosci Res* 50, no. 3 (November 2004): 307–17.

184 Straits Research, *Sleep Market Size, Share & Trends Analysis Report* (2023).

185 American Academy of Sleep Medicine, "One in Three Americans Have Used Electronic Sleep Trackers, Leading to Changed Behavior for Many" (2023).

186 J. E. Ferrie et al., "Sleep Epidemiology—a Rapidly Growing Field," *International Journal of Epidemiology* 40 (2011): 1431–7.

187 C. M. Barnes, "I'll Sleep When I'm Dead: Managing Those Too Busy to Sleep," *Organizational Dynamics* 40, no. 1 (2011): 18–26.

188 R. L. Helmreich, "Culture and Error in Space: Implications from Analog Environments," *Aviat Space Environ Med* 71, suppl. 9 (2000): A133–39, https://www.psy.utexas.edu/psy/helmreich/nasaut.htm.

189 T. Roenneberg et al., "Social Jetlag and Obesity," *Current Biology* 22, no. 10 (2012): 939–43.

190 M. B. Stein et al., "Impairment Associated with Sleep Problems in the Community: Relationship to Physical and Mental Health Comorbidity," *Psychosom Med* 70, no. 8 (October 2008): 913–9.

191 P. M. Krueger and E. M. Friedman, "Sleep Duration in the United States: A Cross-Sectional Population-Based Study," *Am J Epidemiol* 169, no. 9 (May 2009): 1052–63.

192 R. J. Adams et al., "Sleep Health of Australian Adults in 2016: Results of the 2016 Sleep Health Foundation National Survey," *Sleep Health* 3, no. 1 (Feb. 1, 2017): 35–42.

193 M. M. Ohayon, "Epidemiological Overview of Sleep Disorders in the General Population," *Sleep Med Res* 2, no. 1 (2011): 1–9.

194 J. A. Groeger, F. R. H. Zijlstra, and D. J. Dijk, "Sleep Quantity, Sleep Difficulties and Their Perceived Consequences in a Representative Sample of Some 2,000 British Adults," *J Sleep Res* 13 (2004): 359–71.

195 M. Hirshkowitz et al., "National Sleep Foundation's Sleep Time Duration Recommendations: Methodology and Results Summary," *Sleep Health* 1, no. 1 (Mar. 1, 2015): 40–43.

196 N. F. Watson et al., "Recommended Amount of Sleep for a Healthy Adult: A Joint Consensus Statement of the American Academy of Sleep Medicine and Sleep Research Society," *American Academy of Sleep Medicine and Sleep Research Society* 38, no. 6 (2015): 843–4.

197 A. Hirano et al., "DEC2 Modulates Orexin Expression and Regulates Sleep," *Proc Natl Acad Sci USA* 115, no. 13 (Mar. 27, 2018): 3434–39.

198 Y. He et al., "The Transcriptional Repressor DEC2 Regulates Sleep Length in Mammals," *Science* 325, no. 5942 (2009): 866–70.

199 G. Shi et al., "Human Genetics and Sleep Behavior," *Current Opinion in Neurobiology* 44 (2017): 43–49.

200 National Library of Medicine, *Reference SNP (rs) Report—Short Genetic Variations, 2023* (Feb. 20, 2023), rs121912617 RefSNP Report.

201 J. H. Yook et al., "Some Twist of Molecular Circuitry Fast Forwards Overnight Sleep Hours: A Systematic Review of Natural Short Sleepers' Genes," *Cureus* 13, no. 10 (October 2021): e19045.

202 H. P. A. Van Dongen et al., "The Cumulative Cost of Additional Wakefulness: Dose-Response Effects on Neurobehavioral Functions and Sleep Physiology from Chronic Sleep Restriction and Total Sleep Deprivation," *Sleep* 26, no. 2 (2003): 117–26.

203 M. A. St Hilaire et al., "Modeling Neurocognitive Decline and Recovery during Repeated Cycles of Extended Sleep and Chronic Sleep Deficiency," *Sleep* 40, no. 1 (2017).

204 S. Claudio, "The Effects of Polyphasic and Ultrashort Sleep Schedules," in *Why We Nap*, 1st ed., ed. C. Stampi (New York: Springer, 1992), 137–79.

205 C. Stampi, "Polyphasic Sleep Strategies Improve Prolonged Sustained Performance: A Field Study on 99 Sailors," *Work Stress* 3, no. 1 (1989): 41–55.

206 U. N. Sio, P. Monaghan, and T. Ormerod, "Sleep on It, but Only If It Is Difficult: Effects of Sleep on Problem Solving," *Mem Cognit* 41, no. 2 (2013): 159–66.

207 M. P. Walker and E. van der Helm, "Overnight Therapy? The Role of Sleep in Emotional Brain Processing," *Psychol Bull* 135, no. 5 (September 2009): 731–48.

208 C. M. Barnes, "Working in Our Sleep: Sleep and Self-Regulation in Organizations," *Organizational Psychology Review* 2, no. 3 (2012): 234–57.

209 S. Cohen et al., "Sleep Habits and Susceptibility to the Common Cold," *Arch Intern Med* 169, no. 1 (Jan. 12, 2009): 62–67.

210 C. D. Chapman et al., "Acute Sleep Deprivation Increases Food Purchasing in Men," *Obesity* 21, no. 12 (December 2013).

211 S. J. Linton et al., "The Effect of the Work Environment on Future Sleep Disturbances: A Systematic Review," *Sleep Med Rev* 23 (2015): 10–19.

212 M. Van Laethem et al., "Psychosocial Work Characteristics and Sleep Quality: A Systematic Review of Longitudinal and Intervention Research," *Scand J Work Environ Health* 39, no. 6 (2013): 535–49.

213 B. Litwiller et al., "The Relationship between Sleep and Work: A Meta-Analysis," *Journal of Applied Psychology* 102, no. 4 (2017): 682–99.

214 R. J. Davidson, "Anxiety and Affective Style: Role of Prefrontal Cortex and Amygdala," *Biol Psychiatry* 51, no. 1 (2002): 68–80.

215 C. M. Barnes, M. E. Schouten, and E. van de Veen, "Management Educators Are Asleep at the Wheel: Integrating the Topic of Sleep into Management Education," in *Work and Sleep: Research Insights for the Workplace*, 1st ed., eds. J. Barling et al. (New York, NY: Oxford University Press, 2016), 263–77.

216 C. M. Barnes et al., "Too Tired to Inspire or Be Inspired: Sleep Deprivation and Charismatic Leadership," *Journal of Applied Psychology* 101, no. 8 (Aug. 1, 2016): 1191–9.

217 F. Beijamini et al., "Sleep Facilitates Problem Solving with No Additional Gain Through Targeted Memory Reactivation," *Front Behav Neurosci* 15 (Mar. 3, 2021).

218 A. M. Williamson and A. Marie Feyer, "Moderate sleep deprivation produces impairments in cognitive and motor performance equivalent to legally prescribed levels of alcohol intoxication," *Occup Environ Med* 57, no. 10 (2000): 649–55.

219 P. A. Lewis, G. Knoblich, and G. Poe, "How Memory Replay in Sleep Boosts Creative Problem-Solving," *Trends Cogn Sci* 22, no. 6 (June 1, 2018): 491–503.

220 C. M. Barnes et al., "Leader Sleep Devaluation, Employee Sleep, and Unethical Behavior," *Sleep Health* 6, no. 3 (June 1, 2020): 411–417.e5.

221 A. J. Krause et al., "The Sleep-Deprived Human Brain," *Nature Reviews Neuroscience* 18 (2017): 404–18.

222 M. Hafner et al., "Why Sleep Matters—The Economic Costs of Insufficient Sleep: A Cross-Country Comparative Analysis," *Rand Health Q* 6, no. 4 (2017): 11.

223 J. Taillard et al., "Sleep in Normal Aging, Homeostatic and Circadian Regulation and Vulnerability to Sleep Deprivation," *Brain Sciences* 11 (2021).

224 H. Locihová et al., "Effect of the Use of Earplugs and Eye Mask on the Quality of Sleep in Intensive Care Patients: A Systematic Review," *Journal of Sleep Research* 27 (2018).

225 V. Greco et al., "Wearing an Eye Mask during Overnight Sleep Improves Episodic Learning and Alertness," *Sleep* 46, no. 3 (Mar. 9, 2023).

226 C. Cajochen et al., "Evening Exposure to a Light-Emitting Diodes (LED)-Backlit Computer Screen Affects Circadian Physiology and Cognitive Performance," *J Appl Physiol* 110 (2011): 1432–8, http://www.jap.org.

227 B. Wood et al., "Light Level and Duration of Exposure Determine the Impact of Self-Luminous Tablets on Melatonin Suppression," *Appl Ergon* 44, no. 2 (2013): 237–40.

228 E. Matheson and B. L. Hainer, "Insomnia: pharmacologic therapy," *American Family Physician* 96, no. 1 (2017): 29-35.

229 S. Bauducco et al., "A Bidirectional Model of Sleep and Technology Use: A Theoretical Review of How Much, for Whom, and Which Mechanisms," *Sleep Medicine Reviews* 76 (2024).

230 D. Halperin, "Environmental Noise and Sleep Disturbances: A Threat to Health?" *Sleep Science* 7, no. 4 (2014): 209–12.

231 N. S. Zheng et al., "Sleep Patterns and Risk of Chronic Disease as Measured by Long-Term Monitoring with Commercial Wearable Devices in the All of Us Research Program," *Nat Med* 30 (2024).

232 P. M. Maki, N. Panay, and J. A. Simon, "Sleep Disturbance Associated with the Menopause," *Menopause* 31, no. 8 (Aug. 1, 2024).

233 A. Brooks and L. Lack, "A Brief Afternoon Nap Following Nocturnal Sleep Restriction: Which Nap Duration Is Most Recuperative?" *Sleep* 29, no. 6 (2006): 831–40.

234 H. Slama et al., "Afternoon Nap and Bright Light Exposure Improve Cognitive Flexibility Post Lunch," *PLoS One* 10, no. 5 (2015): 1–16.

235 M. Hayashi, A. Masuda, and T. Hori, "The Alerting Effects of Caffeine, Bright Light and Face Washing after a Short Daytime Nap," *Clinical Neurophysiology* 114, no. 12 (2003): 2268–78.

236 L. A. Reyner and J. A. Horne, "Suppression of Sleepiness in Drivers: Combination of Caffeine with a Short Nap," *Psychophysiology* 34 (1997): 721–5.

237 A. Nehlig, "Interindividual Differences in Caffeine Metabolism and Factors Driving Caffeine Consumption," *Pharmacol Rev* 70, no. 2 (2018): 384–411.

238 R. V. Patwardhan et al., "Impaired Elimination of Caffeine by Oral Contraceptive Steroids," *J Lab Clin Med* 95, no. 4 (1980): 603–8.

239 I. O. Ebrahim et al., "Alcohol and Sleep I: Effects on Normal Sleep," *Alcohol Clin Exp Res* 37, no. 4 (2013): 539–49.

240 E. Kuosmanen et al., "How Does Sleep Tracking Influence Your Life?: Experiences from a Longitudinal Field Study with a Wearable Ring," *Proc ACM Hum Comput Interact* 6 (2022): 1–19.

241 K. G. Baron et al., "Orthosomnia: Are Some Patients Taking the Quantified Self Too Far?" *Journal of Clinical Sleep Medicine* 13, no. 2 (2017): 351–4.

242 V. Birrer et al., "Evaluating Reliability in Wearable Devices for Sleep Staging," *NPJ Digital Medicine* 7 (2024).

243 C. Draganich and K. Erdal, "Placebo Sleep Affects Cognitive Functioning," *J Exp Psychol Learn Mem Cogn* 40, no. 3 (2014): 857–64.

244 D. Gavriloff et al., "Sham Sleep Feedback Delivered via Actigraphy Biases Daytime Symptom Reports in People with Insomnia: Implications for Insomnia Disorder and Wearable Devices," *J Sleep Res* 27, no. 6 (2018).

245 D. Rae et al., "Wearables That Track Sleep: The Effect of Sham Sleep Feedback on Sleep Quality, Mood and Daytime Functioning," in Oral Session 12, 27th Congress of the European Sleep Research Society, September 24–27, 2024, Seville, Spain (2024), 41.

246 T. S. Church et al., "Trends over 5 Decades in US Occupation-Related Physical Activity and Their Associations with Obesity," *PLoS One* 6, no. 5 (2011).

247 *Economist*, "AI Is Not Yet Killing Jobs" (June 2023).

248 A. L. Gremaud et al., "Gamifying Accelerometer Use Increases Physical Activity Levels of Sedentary Office Workers," *J Am Heart Assoc* 7, no. 13 (July 1, 2018).

249 R. M. Panicker and B. Chandrasekaran, "'Wearables on Vogue': A Scoping Review on Wearables on Physical Activity and Sedentary Behavior during COVID-19 Pandemic," *Sport Sciences for Health* 18 (2022): 641–57.

250 R. Guthold et al., "Worldwide Trends in Insufficient Physical Activity from 2001 to 2016: A Pooled Analysis of 358 Population-Based Surveys with 1.9 Million Participants," *Lancet Glob Health* 6, no. 10 (Oct. 1, 2018): e1077–86.

251 J. A. McVeigh et al., "Objectively Measured Patterns of Sedentary Time and Physical Activity in Young Adults of the Raine Study Cohort," *International Journal of Behavioral Nutrition and Physical Activity* 13, (Mar. 24, 2016).

252 U. Ekelund et al., "Dose-Response Associations between Accelerometry Measured Physical Activity and Sedentary Time and All Cause Mortality: Systematic Review and Harmonised Meta-Analysis," *BMJ* 366 (2019).

253 C. Bouchard, S. N. Blair, and P. T. Katzmarzyk, "Less Sitting, More Physical Activity, or Higher Fitness?" *Mayo Clin Proc* 90, no. 11 (2015): 1533–40.

254 F. C. Bull et al., "World Health Organization 2020 Guidelines on Physical Activity and Sedentary Behaviour," *Br J Sports Med* 54, no. 24 (2020): 1451–62.

255 J. D. Akins et al., "Inactivity Induces Resistance to the Metabolic Benefits Following Acute Exercise," *J Appl Physiol* 126, no. 4 (2019): 1088–94.

256 L. Zhai, Y. Zhang, and D. Zhang, "Sedentary Behaviour and the Risk of Depression: A Meta-Analysis," *Br J Sports Med* 49, no. 11 (2015): 705–9.

257 A. Dėdelė et al., "Perceived Stress among Different Occupational Groups and the Interaction with Sedentary Behaviour," *Int J Environ Res Public Health* 16, no. 23 (Nov. 20, 2019).

258 A. M. Newsome et al., "2024 ACSM Worldwide Fitness Trends: Future Directions of the Health and Fitness Industry Apply It!" *ACSM's Health & Fitness Journal* 28, no. 1 (2024): 14–26.

259 M. Yin et al., "Is Low-Volume High-Intensity Interval Training a Time-Efficient Strategy to Improve Cardiometabolic Health and Body Composition? A Meta-Analysis," *Applied Physiology, Nutrition and Metabolism* 49 (2024): 273–92.

260 M. Flockhart et al., "Excessive Exercise Training Causes Mitochondrial Functional Impairment and Decreases Glucose Tolerance in Healthy Volunteers," *Cell Metab* 33 (2021): 957–70.

261 T. Martikainen et al., "Effects of Curtailed Sleep on Cardiac Stress Biomarkers Following High-Intensity Exercise," *Mol Metab* 58 (Apr. 1, 2022).

262 S. Lamon et al., "The Effect of Acute Sleep Deprivation on Skeletal Muscle Protein Synthesis and the Hormonal Environment," *Physiol Rep* 9, no. 1 (Jan. 1, 2021).

263 M. Pearce et al., "Association between Physical Activity and Risk of Depression: A Systematic Review and Meta-Analysis," *JAMA Psychiatry* 79 (2022): 550–9.

264 M. Hallgren et al., "Passive and Mentally-Active Sedentary Behaviors and Incident Major Depressive Disorder: A 13-Year Cohort Study," *J Affect Disord* 241 (2018): 579–85.

265 M. Hallgren et al., "Cross-Sectional and Prospective Relationships of Passive and Mentally Active Sedentary Behaviours and Physical Activity with Depression," *British Journal of Psychiatry* 217, no. 2 (Aug. 1, 2020): 413–19.

266 N. L. Spartano et al., "Association of Accelerometer-Measured Physical Activity and Sedentary Time with Epigenetic Markers of Aging," *Med Sci Sports Exerc* 55, no. 2 (Feb. 1, 2023): 264–72.

267 B. Del Pozo Cruz et al., "Association of Daily Step Count and Intensity with Incident Dementia in 78,430 Adults Living in the UK," *JAMA Neurol* 79, no. 10 (Oct. 1, 2022): 1059–63.

268 K. S. Hall et al., "Systematic Review of the Prospective Association of Daily Step Counts with Risk of Mortality, Cardiovascular Disease, and Dysglycemia," *International Journal of Behavioral Nutrition and Physical Activity* 17, no. 1 (June 20, 2020).

269 C. Tudor-Locke et al., "How Many Steps/Day Are Enough? For Adults," *International Journal of Behavioral Nutrition and Physical Activity* 8, no. 1 (2011): 79.

270 World Health Organization, *WHO Guidelines on Physical Activity and Sedentary Behaviour* (2020).

271 S. Dattani et al., "Life Expectancy," *Our World in Data* (2023).

272 F. Yin et al., "Mitochondrial Function in Ageing: Coordination with Signalling and Transcriptional Pathways," *Journal of Physiology* 594 (2016): 2025–42.

273 K. S. Mølmen, N. W. Almquist, and Ø. Skattebo, "Effects of Exercise Training on Mitochondrial and Capillary Growth in Human Skeletal Muscle: A Systematic Review and Meta-Regression," *Sports Med* 55 (Oct. 10, 2024).

274 D. J. Bishop, C. Granata, and N. Eynon, "Can We Optimise the Exercise Training Prescription to Maximise Improvements in Mitochondria Function and Content?" *Biochimica et Biophysica Acta—General Subjects* 1840 (2014): 1266–75.

275 P. J. Adhihetty et al., "Plasticity of Skeletal Muscle Mitochondria in Response to Contractile Activity," *Experimental Physiology* 88 (2003): 99–107.

276 Y. Netz, "Is the Comparison between Exercise and Pharmacologic Treatment of Depression in the Clinical Practice Guideline of the American College of Physicians Evidence-Based?" *Front Pharmacol* 8 (May 15, 2017).

277 G. O'Donovan et al., "Association of 'Weekend Warrior' and Other Leisure Time Physical Activity Patterns with Risks for All-Cause, Cardiovascular Disease, and Cancer Mortality," *JAMA Internal Medicine* 177 (2017): 335–42.

278 A. Doherty et al., "Large Scale Population Assessment of Physical Activity Using Wrist Worn Accelerometers: The UK Biobank Study," *PLoS One* 12, no. 2 (Feb. 1, 2017).

279 G. O'Donovan et al., "Associations of the 'Weekend Warrior' Physical Activity Pattern with Mild Dementia: Findings from the Mexico City Prospective Study," *Br J Sports Med* 59, no. 5 (2025): 325–32.

280 E. Tønnessen et al., "Maximal Aerobic Capacity in the Winter-Olympics Endurance Disciplines Olympic-Medal Benchmarks for the Time Period 1990–2013," *International Journal of Sports Physiology and Performance* 10 (2015): 835–9.

281 K. Mandsager et al., "Association of Cardiorespiratory Fitness with Long-term Mortality among Adults Undergoing Exercise Treadmill Testing," *JAMA Netw Open* 1, no. 6 (Oct. 5, 2018): e183605.

282 R. Ross et al., "Importance of Assessing Cardiorespiratory Fitness in Clinical Practice: A Case for Fitness as a Clinical Vital Sign: A Scientific Statement from the American Heart Association," *Circulation* 134 (2016): e653–99.

283 J. A. Laukkanen, N. M. Isiozor, and S. K. Kunutsor, "Objectively Assessed Cardiorespiratory Fitness and All-Cause Mortality Risk: An Updated Meta-Analysis of 37 Cohort Studies Involving 2,258,029 Participants," *Mayo Clin Proc* 97, no. 6 (2022): 1054–73.

284 K. J. Gries et al., "Cardiovascular and Skeletal Muscle Health with Lifelong Exercise," *J Appl Physiol* 125, no. 5 (2018): 1636–45.

285 Apple Inc., "Using Apple Watch to Estimate Cardio Fitness with VO2 Max" (2021).

286 P. Düking, B. Van Hooren, and B. Sperlich, "Assessment of Peak Oxygen Uptake with a Smartwatch and Its Usefulness for Training of Runners," *Int J Sports Med* 43, no. 7 (June 1, 2022): 642–7.

287 Firstbeat Technologies Ltd., "Automated Fitness Level (VO2 Max) Estimation with Heart Rate and Speed Data," Whitepaper (2014), 1–9.

288 C. Bouchard et al., "Genetics of Aerobic and Anaerobic Performances," *Exerc Sport Sci Rev* 20 (1992): 27–58.

289 D. Laury and A. Tehrany, "VO2 Max Improvement of 96% in a Non-Elite Recreational Athlete over 24 Months," *Surgery Journal* 5, no. 1 (April 2019): e25–7.

290 J. Burtscher et al., "The Impact of Training on the Loss of Cardiorespiratory Fitness in Aging Masters Endurance Athletes," *International Journal of Environmental Research and Public Health* 19 (2022).

291 Z. Milanović, G. Sporiš, and M. Weston, "Effectiveness of High-Intensity Interval Training (HIT) and Continuous Endurance Training for VO2 Max Improvements: A Systematic Review and Meta-Analysis of Controlled Trials," *Sports Medicine* 45 (2015): 1469–81.

292 R. S. Metcalfe et al., "Towards the Minimal Amount of Exercise for Improving Metabolic Health: Beneficial Effects of Reduced-Exertion High-Intensity Interval Training," *Eur J Appl Physiol* 112, no. 7 (July 2012): 2767–75.

293 E. M. Jenkins et al., "Do Stair Climbing Exercise 'Snacks' Improve Cardiorespiratory Fitness?," *Appl Physiol Nutr Metab* 44, no. 6 (January 2019): 681–4.

294 M. E. Francois et al., "'Exercise Snacks' before Meals: A Novel Strategy to Improve Glycaemic Control in Individuals with Insulin Resistance," *Diabetologia* 57, no. 7 (2014): 1437–45.

295 E. Stamatakis et al., "Association of Wearable Device-Measured Vigorous Intermittent Lifestyle Physical Activity with Mortality," *Nat Med* 28, no. 12 (Dec. 1, 2022): 2521–9.

296 R. Martland et al., "Can High-Intensity Interval Training Improve Mental Health Outcomes in the General Population and Those with Physical Illnesses? A Systematic Review and Meta-Analysis," *British Journal of Sports Medicine* 56 (2022): 279–91.

297 D. G. Blackmore et al., "Long-Term Improvement in Hippocampal-Dependent Learning Ability in Healthy, Aged Individuals Following High Intensity Interval Training," *Aging Dis* (2024).

298 D. J. Wilkinson, M. Piasecki, and P. J. Atherton, "The Age-Related Loss of Skeletal Muscle Mass and Function: Measurement and Physiology of Muscle Fibre Atrophy and Muscle Fibre Loss in Humans," *Ageing Res Rev* 47 (November 2018): 123–32.

299 E. G. Artero et al., "Effects of Muscular Strength on Cardiovascular Risk Factors and Prognosis," *Journal of Cardiopulmonary Rehabilitation and Prevention* 32 (2012): 351–8.

300 P. Srikanthan and A. S. Karlamangla, "Muscle Mass Index as a Predictor of Longevity in Older Adults," *American Journal of Medicine* 127, no. 6 (2014): 547–53.

301 K. F. Reid and R. A. Fielding, "Skeletal Muscle Power: A Critical Determinant of Physical Functioning in Older Adults," *Exerc Sport Sci Rev* 40, no. 1 (January 2012): 4–12.

302 E. L. Cadore et al., "Multicomponent Exercises Including Muscle Power Training Enhance Muscle Mass, Power Output, and Functional Outcomes in Institutionalized Frail Nonagenarians," *Age* 36, no. 2 (2014): 773–85.

303 Strava, *Year in Sport—the Trend Report* (Sep. 2023).

304 S. Schnall et al., "Social Support and the Perception of Geographical Slant," *J Exp Soc Psychol* 44, no. 5 (September 2008): 1246–55.

305 K. Sick, S. Rollo, and H. Prapavessis, "Exploring the Relationship between Adults' Perceptions of Sedentary Behaviours and Psychological Stress: Is Your Mindset Stressing You Out?" *Int J Sport Exerc Psychol* 20, no. 4 (2022): 1208–24.

306 C. A. Monteiro et al., "The Food System," *World Nutrition* 7, no. 3 (2016).

307 C. A. Monteiro and G. Cannon, "Ultra-Processed Foods and Food Addiction," in *Food and Addiction: A Comprehensive Handbook*, 2nd ed., eds. A. N. Gearhardt et al. (Oxford: Oxford University Press, 2024), 289.

308 K. Whelan et al., "Ultra-Processed Foods and Food Additives in Gut Health and Disease," *Nat Rev Gastroenterol Hepatol* 21, no. 6 (2024): 406–27.

309 P. E. Taneri et al., "Association between Ultra-Processed Food Intake and All-Cause Mortality: A Systematic Review and Meta-Analysis," *American Journal of Epidemiology* 191 (2022): 1323–35.

310 M. Askari et al., "Ultra-Processed Food and the Risk of Overweight and Obesity: A Systematic Review and Meta-Analysis of Observational Studies," *Int J Obes* 44, no. 10 (Oct. 1, 2020): 2080–91.

311 J. M. Poti, B. Braga, and B. Qin, "Ultra-Processed Food Intake and Obesity: What Really Matters for Health-Processing or Nutrient Content?" *Current Obesity Reports* 6 (2017): 420–31.

312 M. I. Almarshad et al., "Relationship between Ultra-Processed Food Consumption and Risk of Diabetes Mellitus: A Mini-Review," *Nutrients* 14, no. 12 (June 7, 2022).

313 S. L. Canhada et al., "Association between Ultra-Processed Food Consumption and the Incidence of Type 2 Diabetes: The ELSA-Brasil Cohort," *Diabetol Metab Syndr* 15, no. 1 (Nov. 15, 2023).

314 M. Li and Z. Shi, "Ultra-Processed Food Consumption Associated with Incident Hypertension Among Chinese Adults—Results from China Health and Nutrition Survey 1997–2015," *Nutrients* 14, no. 22 (Nov. 11, 2022).

315 N. G. Gonçalves et al., "Association between Consumption of Ultraprocessed Foods and Cognitive Decline," *JAMA Neurol* 80, no. 2 (Feb. 1, 2023): 142–50.

316 C. Patikorn et al., "Effects of Ketogenic Diet on Health Outcomes: An Umbrella Review of Meta-Analyses of Randomized Clinical Trials," *BMC Med* 21, no. 1 (May 25, 2023).

317 G. Taubes, *Why We Get Fat: And What to Do About It* (New York: Alfred A. Knopf, 2011).

318 K. D. Hall et al., "Energy Expenditure and Body Composition Changes after an Isocaloric Ketogenic Diet in Overweight and Obese Men," *American Journal of Clinical Nutrition* 104, no. 2 (Aug. 1, 2016): 324–33.

319 K. D. Hall, "A Review of the Carbohydrate-Insulin Model of Obesity," *Eur J Clin Nutr* 71, no. 3 (Mar. 1, 2017): 323–6.

320 K. D. Hall, S. J. Guyenet, and R. L. Leibel, "The Carbohydrate-Insulin Model of Obesity Is Difficult to Reconcile with Current Evidence," *JAMA Internal Medicine* 178 (2018): 1103–5.

321 D. S. Ludwig et al., "Competing Paradigms of Obesity Pathogenesis: Energy Balance versus Carbohydrate-Insulin Models," *Eur J Clin Nutr* 76, no. 9 (Sep. 1, 2022): 1209–21.

322 A. P. Shukla et al., "Food Order Has a Significant Impact on Postprandial Glucose and Insulin Levels," *Diabetes Care* 38 (2015): e98–9.

323 A. Ceriello and S. Genovese, "Atherogenicity of Postprandial Hyperglycemia and Lipotoxicity," *Reviews in Endocrine and Metabolic Disorders* 17 (2016): 111–6.

324 L. Monnier, C. Colette, and D. R. Owens, "Glycemic Variability: The Third Component of the Dysglycemia in Diabetes. Is It Important? How to Measure It?" *Journal of Diabetes Science and Technology* 2 (2008), https://www.journalofdst.org.

325 A. Bellini et al., "Effects of Different Exercise Strategies to Improve Postprandial Glycemia in Healthy Individuals," *Med Sci Sports Exerc* 53, no. 7 (2021): 1334–44.

326 M. Rafii et al., "Dietary Protein Requirement of Female Adults >65 Years Determined by the Indicator Amino Acid Oxidation Technique Is Higher than Current Recommendations," *Journal of Nutrition* 145, no. 1 (2015): 18–24.

327 M. Rafii et al., "Dietary Protein Requirement of Men >65 Years Old Determined by the Indicator Amino Acid Oxidation Technique Is Higher than the Current Estimated Average Requirement," *Journal of Nutrition* 146, no. 4 (Apr. 1, 2015): 681–7.

328 S. M. Phillips, "Current Concepts and Unresolved Questions in Dietary Protein Requirements and Supplements in Adults," *Front Nutr* 4 (May 2017): 1–10.

329 D. A. Traylor, S. H. M. Gorissen, and S. M. Phillips, "Perspective: Protein Requirements and Optimal Intakes in Aging: Are We Ready to Recommend More than the Recommended Daily Allowance?" *Advances in Nutrition* 9, no. 3 (2018): 171–82.

330 R. R. Wolfe et al., "Optimizing Protein Intake in Adults: Interpretation and Application of the Recommended Dietary Allowance Compared with the Acceptable Macronutrient Distribution Range," *Advances in Nutrition* 8, no. 2 (Mar. 15, 2017): 266–75.

331 D. Paddon-Jones et al., "Protein, Weight Management, and Satiety," *Am J Clin Nutr* 87, no. 5 (2008): 1558–61.

332 M. C. Devries et al., "Changes in Kidney Function Do Not Differ between Healthy Adults Consuming Higher-Compared with Lower- or Normal-Protein Diets: A Systematic Review and Meta-Analysis," *Journal of Nutrition* 148, no. 11 (Nov. 1, 2018): 1760–75.

333 S. M. Phillips and L. J. C. Van Loon, "Dietary Protein for Athletes: From Requirements to Optimum Adaptation," *J Sports Sci* 29, suppl. 1 (2011).

334 S. Adhikari et al., "Protein Quality in Perspective: A Review of Protein Quality Metrics and Their Applications," *Nutrients* 14, no. 5 (Feb. 23, 2022).

335 A. K. Roberts et al., "SWAP-MEAT Athlete (Study with Appetizing Plant-Food, Meat Eating Alternatives Trial)—Investigating the Impact of Three Different Diets on Recreational Athletic Performance: A Randomized Crossover Trial," *Nutr J* 21, no. 1 (Nov. 16, 2022).

336 J. Trommelen et al., "The Anabolic Response to Protein Ingestion during Recovery from Exercise Has No Upper Limit in Magnitude and Duration in Vivo in Humans," *Cell Rep Med* 4, no. 12 (Dec. 19, 2023).

337 A. G. Liu et al., "A Healthy Approach to Dietary Fats: Understanding the Science and Taking Action to Reduce Consumer Confusion," *Nutrition Journal* 16 (2017).

338 M. A. Islam et al., "Trans Fatty Acids and Lipid Profile: A Serious Risk Factor to Cardiovascular Disease, Cancer and Diabetes," *Diabetes and Metabolic Syndrome: Clinical Research and Reviews* 13, no. 2 (2019): 1643–7.

339 I. Djuricic and P. C. Calder, "Beneficial Outcomes of Omega-6 and Omega-3 Polyunsaturated Fatty Acids on Human Health: An Update for 2021," *Nutrients* 13, no. 7 (July 1, 2021).

340 F. Bellisle, R. McDevitt, and A. M. Prentice, "Meal Frequency and Energy Balance," *British Journal of Nutrition* 77, suppl. 1 (April 1997): S57–70.

341 X. Yuan et al., "Effect of Intermittent Fasting Diet on Glucose and Lipid Metabolism and Insulin Resistance in Patients with Impaired Glucose and Lipid Metabolism: A Systematic Review and Meta-Analysis," *International Journal of Endocrinology* 2022 (2022).

342 Q. Zhang et al., "Intermittent Fasting versus Continuous Calorie Restriction: Which Is Better for Weight Loss?" *Nutrients* 14, no. 9 (Apr. 24, 2022).

343 Y. Chang et al., "Time-Restricted Eating Improves Health because of Energy Deficit and Circadian Rhythm: A Systematic Review and Meta-Analysis," *iScience* 27, no. 2 (Jan. 26, 2024).

344 B. J. Schoenfeld et al., "Body Composition Changes Associated with Fasted versus Non-Fasted Aerobic Exercise," *J Int Soc Sports Nutr* 11, no. 1 (2014).

345 H. Zouhal et al., "Exercise Training and Fasting: Current Insights," *Open Access Journal of Sports Medicine* 11 (2020): 1–28.

346 J. O'Leary, C. Georgeaux-Healy, and L. Serpell, "The Impact of Continuous Calorie Restriction and Fasting on Cognition in Adults Without Eating Disorders," *Nutr Rev* 83 (2025): 146–59.

347 M. V. Deligiorgi, C. Liapi, and D. T. Trafalis, "How Far Are We from Prescribing Fasting as Anticancer Medicine?" *International Journal of Molecular Sciences* 21 (2020): 1–30.

348 D. A. Lowe et al., "Effects of Time-Restricted Eating on Weight Loss and Other Metabolic Parameters in Women and Men with Overweight and Obesity: The TREAT Randomized Clinical Trial," *JAMA Intern Med* 180, no. 11 (Nov. 1, 2020): 1491–9.

349 G. M. Tinsley and A. Paoli, "Time-Restricted Eating and Age-Related Muscle Loss," *Aging* 11, no. 20 (2019): 8741–2.

350 K. A. Varady et al., "Debunking the Myths of Intermittent Fasting," *Nat Rev Endocrinol* 20 (2024): 503–4.

351 M. Franzago et al., "Chrono-Nutrition: Circadian Rhythm and Personalized Nutrition," *International Journal of Molecular Sciences* 24 (2023).

352 R. Chamorro et al., "When Should I Eat: A Circadian View on Food Intake and Metabolic Regulation," *Acta Physiologica* 237 (2023).

353 P. Lewis et al., "Food as a Circadian Time Cue—Evidence from Human Studies," *Nat Rev Endocrinol* 16, no. 4 (2020): 213–23.

354 C. Gu et al., "Metabolic Effects of Late Dinner in Healthy Volunteers—A Randomized Crossover Clinical Trial," *Journal of Clinical Endocrinology and Metabolism* 105, no. 8 (Aug. 1, 2020): 2789–802.

355 E. Tajiri et al., "Effects of Sleep Restriction on Food Intake and Appetite under Free-Living Conditions: A Randomized Crossover Trial," *Appetite* 189 (Oct. 1, 2023).

356 R. M. Tucker et al., "The Influence of Sleep on Human Taste Function and Perception: A Systematic Review," *Journal of Sleep Research* 34 (2024).

357 Grand View Research, *Nutritional Supplements Market Size, Share & Trends Analysis* (2003).

358 R. E. Wierzejska, "Dietary Supplements—For Whom? The Current State of Knowledge about the Health Effects of Selected Supplement Use," *International Journal of Environmental Research and Public Health* 18 (2021).

359 C. Weikert et al., "Versorgungsstatus mit Vitaminen und Mineralstoffen bei veganer Ernährungsweise," *Dtsch Arztebl Int* 117, nos. 35–36 (Aug. 31, 2020): 575–82.

360 A. Prentice, "Vitamin D Deficiency: A Global Perspective," *Nutrition Reviews* 66 (2008).

361 E. Wooltorton, "Too Much of a Good Thing? Toxic Effects of Vitamin and Mineral Supplements," *CMAJ* 169, no. 1 (2003): 47–48.

362 Y. Dotan et al., "Decision Analysis Supports the Paradigm That Indiscriminate Supplementation of Vitamin E Does More Harm than Good," *Arterioscler Thromb Vasc Biol* 29, no. 9 (September 2009): 1304–9.

363 B. G. Brown et al., "Simvastatin and Niacin, Antioxidant Vitamins, or the Combination for the Prevention of Coronary Disease," *N Engl J Med* 345, no. 22 (2001): 1583.

364 J. Mah and T. Pitre, "Oral Magnesium Supplementation for Insomnia in Older Adults: A Systematic Review and Meta-Analysis," *BMC Complement Med Ther* 21, no. 1 (Apr. 17, 2021).

365 M. J. Breus et al., "Effectiveness of Magnesium Supplementation on Sleep Quality and Mood for Adults with Poor Sleep Quality: A Randomized Double-Blind Placebo-Controlled Crossover Pilot Trial," *Med Res Arch* 12, no. 7 (2024).

366 N. A. Revankar and P. S. Negi, "Biotics: An Emerging Food Supplement for Health Improvement in the Era of Immune Modulation," *Nutr Clin Pract* 39, no. 2 (2024): 311–29.

367   J. Antonio et al., "Common Questions and Misconceptions about Creatine Supplementation: What Does the Scientific Evidence Really Show?" *J Int Soc Sports Nutr* 18, no. 1 (Feb. 8, 2021).

368   R. B. Kreider et al., "International Society of Sports Nutrition Position Stand: Safety and Efficacy of Creatine Supplementation in Exercise, Sport, and Medicine," *Journal of the International Society of Sports Nutrition* 14 (2017).

369   Z. Wang et al., "Effects of Creatine Supplementation and Resistance Training on Muscle Strength Gains in Adults <50 Years of Age: A Systematic Review and Meta-Analysis," *Nutrients* 16, no. 21 (Oct. 28, 2024): 3665.

370   D. Van Bavel, R. de Moraes, and E. Tibirica, "Effects of Dietary Supplementation with Creatine on Homocysteinemia and Systemic Microvascular Endothelial Function in Individuals Adhering to Vegan Diets," *Fundam Clin Pharmacol* 33, no. 4 (Aug. 1, 2019): 428–40.

371   M. Kaviani, K. Shaw, and P. D. Chilibeck, "Benefits of Creatine Supplementation for Vegetarians Compared to Omnivorous Athletes: A Systematic Review," *Int J Environ Res Public Health* 17, no. 9 (Apr. 27, 2020).

372   S. E. Berry et al., "Human Postprandial Responses to Food and Potential for Precision Nutrition," *Nat Med* 26, no. 6 (June 1, 2020): 964–73.

373   C. Celis-Morales et al., "Effect of Personalized Nutrition on Health-Related Behaviour Change: Evidence from the Food4Me European Randomized Controlled Trial," *Int J Epidemiol* 46, no. 2 (2017): 578–88.

374   J. M. Ordovas et al., "Personalised Nutrition and Health," *BMJ* [Internet] 361 (2018): 1–7.

375   K. M. Bermingham et al., "Effects of a Personalized Nutrition Program on Cardiometabolic Health: A Randomized Controlled Trial," *Nat Med* 30, no. 7 (July 1, 2024): 1888–97.

376   E. Diener and M. Y. Chan, "Happy People Live Longer: Subjective Well-Being Contributes to Health and Longevity," *Appl Psychol Health Well Being* 3, no. 1 (2011): 1–43.

377   M. Pollan, "Unhappy Meals," *New York Times Magazine* (Jan. 28, 2007).

378   Health and Safety Executive, *Trends in Work-Related Ill Health and Workplace Injury* (London, 2022).

379   American Psychological Association, *2023 Work in America Survey* (2023).

380   K. Shah and D. Tomlinson, "Work Experiences: Changes in the Subjective Experience of Work" (2021).

381   A. Felstead et al., "Skills and Employment Survey, 2017" (2019).

382   J. Brassey et al., "Addressing Employee Burnout: Are You Solving the Right Problem?" (2022).

383   A. J. Crum et al., "Evaluation of the 'Rethink Stress' Mindset Intervention: A Metacognitive Approach to Changing Mindsets," *J Exp Psychol Gen* (Sep. 18, 2023).

384   J. P. Jamieson et al., "Optimizing Stress Responses with Reappraisal and Mindset Interventions: An Integrated Model," *Anxiety Stress Coping* 31, no. 3 (May 4, 2018): 245–61.

385   C. Happer and G. Philo, "The Role of the Media in the Construction of Public Belief and Social Change," *Journal of Social and Political Psychology* 1, no. 1 (2013): 321–36.

386   R. S. Lazarus and S. F. Folkman, *Stress, Appraisal, and Coping* (New York: Springer, 1984).

387   C. L. Park and S. Folkman, "Meaning in the Context of Stress and Coping," *Review of General Psychology* 1, no. 2 (1997): 115–44.

388   S. C. Hayes et al., "Experiential Avoidance and Behavioral Disorders: A Functional Dimensional Approach to Diagnosis and Treatment," *J Consult Clin Psychol* 64, no. 6 (1996): 1152–68.

389   K. E. Weick and K. M. Sutcliffe, "Mindfulness and the Quality of Organizational Attention," *Organization Science* 17, no. 4 (2006): 514–24.

390   D. A. Moore and P. J. Healy, "The Trouble with Overconfidence," *Psychol Rev* 115, no. 2 (April 2008): 502–17.

391   L. M. Shin and I. Liberzon, "The Neurocircuitry of Fear, Stress, and Anxiety Disorders," *Neuropsychopharmacology* 35, no. 1 (January 2010): 169–91.

392   A. F. T. Arnsten, "Stress Signalling Pathways That Impair Prefrontal Cortex Structure and Function," *Nat Rev Neurosci* 10, no. 6 (2009): 410–22.

393   C. A. Moodie et al., "The Neural Bases of Cognitive Emotion Regulation: The Roles of Strategy and Intensity," *Cogn Affect Behav Neurosci* 20, no. 2 (Apr. 1, 2020): 387–407.

394   A. F. T. Arnsten, "Stress Weakens Prefrontal Networks: Molecular Insults to Higher Cognition." *Nat Neurosci* 18, no. 10 (Oct. 28, 2015): 1376–85.

395   E. J. Kim, B. Pellman, and J. J. Kim, "Stress Effects on the Hippocampus: A Critical Review," *Learning & Memory* 22, no. 9 (2015): 411–6.

396   G. Aguilera, "HPA Axis Responsiveness to Stress: Implications for Healthy Aging," *Exp Gerontol* 46, nos. 2–3 (2011): 90–5.

397 J. P. Herman et al., "Regulation of the Hypothalamic-Pituitary-Adrenocortical Stress Response," *Compr Physiol* 6, no. 2 (Mar. 15, 2016): 603–21.

398 C. Tsigos and G. P. Chrousos, "Hypothalamic-Pituitary-Adrenal Axis, Neuroendocrine Factors and Stress," *J Psychosom Res* 53 (2002): 865–71.

399 D. S. Goldstein, "Adrenal Responses to Stress," *Cell Mol Neurobiol* 30, no. 8 (2010): 1433–40.

400 R. M. Sapolsky, L. M. Romero, and A. U. Munck, "How Do Glucocorticoids Influence Stress Responses? Integrating Permissive, Suppressive, Stimulatory, and Preparative Actions," *Endocr Rev* 21, no. 1 (2000): 55–89.

401 J. K. Gjerstad, S. L. Lightman, and F. Spiga, "Role of Glucocorticoid Negative Feedback in the Regulation of HPA Axis Pulsatility," *Stress* 21, no. 5 (2018): 403–16.

402 M. B. Hargrove, D. L. Nelson, and C. L. Cooper, "Generating Eustress by Challenging Employees. Helping People Savor Their Work," *Organ Dyn* 42, no. 1 (Jan. 2013): 61–69.

403 B. S. McEwen, "Protective and Damaging Effects of Stress Mediators," *New England Journal of Medicine* 338, no. 3 (1998): 171–9.

404 T. Saunders et al., "The Effect of Stress Inoculation Training on Anxiety and Performance," *Journal of Occupational Health Psychology* 1 (1996).

405 C. Peterson and M. E. P. Seligman, *Character Strengths and Virtues: A Handbook and Classification* (Oxford: Oxford University Press, 2004).

406 T. Yan et al., "Development of an Evidence-Based, Theory-Driven, and Culturally Appropriate Character Strengths-Based Intervention for Breast Cancer Patients, Following the Medical Research Council Framework," *Supportive Care in Cancer* 31, no. 1 (Dec. 16, 2022).

407 L. Wagner et al., "Character Strengths and PERMA: Investigating the Relationships of Character Strengths with a Multidimensional Framework of Well-Being," *Appl Res Qual Life* 15, no. 2 (Apr. 1, 2020): 307–28.

408 R. M. Niemiec, "Finding the Golden Mean: The Overuse, Underuse, and Optimal Use of Character Strengths," *Couns Psychol Q* 32, nos. 3–4 (Oct. 2, 2019): 453–71.

409 F. D. Fincham and K. M. Cain, "Learned Helplessness in Humans: A Developmental Analysis," *Developmental Review* 6 (1986): 301–33.

410 A. W. Brooks, "Get Excited: Reappraising Pre-Performance Anxiety as Excitement," *J Exp Psychol Gen* 143, no. 3 (2014): 1144–58.

411 A. J. Crum, P. Salovey, and S. Achor, "Rethinking Stress: The Role of Mindsets in Determining the Stress Response," *J Pers Soc Psychol* 104, no. 4 (2013): 716–33.

412 J. P. Jamieson et al., "Turning the Knots in Your Stomach into Bows: Reappraising Arousal Improves Performance on the GRE," *J Exp Soc Psychol* 46, no. 1 (January 2010): 208–12.

413 A. Crum, "Rethink Stress Intervention," *Stanford University Mind & Body Lab* (2024).

414 A. J. Crum et al., "The Role of Stress Mindset in Shaping Cognitive, Emotional, and Physiological Responses to Challenging and Threatening Stress," *Anxiety Stress Coping* 30, no. 4 (July 4, 2017): 379–95.

415 J. W. Y. Kam et al., "A Brief Reappraisal Intervention Leads to Durable Affective Benefits," *Emotion* 24, no. 7 (2024): 1676–88.

416 J. Song, B. F. Jeronimus, and A. J. Fisher, "Sleep, Event Appraisal, and Affect: An Ecological Momentary Assessment Study," *J Affect Disord* 361 (Sep. 15, 2024): 376–82.

417 Y. C. Chen et al., "Habitual Physical Activity Mediates the Acute Exercise-Induced Modulation of Anxiety-Related Amygdala Functional Connectivity," *Sci Rep* 9, no. 1 (2019): 1–12.

418 E. Childs and H. de Wit, "Regular Exercise Is Associated with Emotional Resilience to Acute Stress in Healthy Adults," *Front Physiol* 5 (May 5, 2014): 1–7.

419 B. von Haaren et al., "Does a 20-Week Aerobic Exercise Training Programme Increase Our Capabilities to Buffer Real-Life Stressors? A Randomized, Controlled Trial Using Ambulatory Assessment," *Eur J Appl Physiol* 116, no. 2 (Feb. 1, 2016): 383–94.

420 I. Ensari et al., "Testing the Cross-Stressor Hypothesis under Real-World Conditions: Exercise as a Moderator of the Association between Momentary Anxiety and Cardiovascular Responses," *J Behav Med* 43, no. 6 (Dec. 1, 2020): 989–1001.

421 N. T. Van Dam et al., "Mind the Hype: A Critical Evaluation and Prescriptive Agenda for Research on Mindfulness and Meditation," *Perspectives on Psychological Science* 13, no. 1 (Jan. 1, 2018): 36–61.

422 M. Goyal et al., "Meditation Programs for Psychological Stress and Well-Being: A Systematic Review and Meta-Analysis," *JAMA Intern Med* 174, no. 3 (2014): 357–68.

423 J. Galante et al., "Systematic Review and Individual Participant Data Meta-Analysis of Randomized Controlled Trials Assessing Mindfulness-Based Programs for Mental Health Promotion," *Nature Mental Health* 1, no. 7 (July 10, 2023): 462–76.

424 C. R. Pernet et al., "Mindfulness Related Changes in Grey Matter: A Systematic Review and Meta-Analysis," *Brain Imaging Behav* 15 (2021): 2720–30.

425 S. Siew and J. Yu, "Mindfulness-Based Randomized Controlled Trials Led to Brain Structural Changes: An Anatomical Likelihood Meta-Analysis," *Sci Rep* 13, no. 1 (Oct. 27, 2023).

426 Editorial, "Mindfulness Research Needs an Intervention," *Nature Mental Health* 1, no. 7 (July 10, 2023): 437–38.

427 C. Strauss et al., "Mindfulness-Based Interventions for People Diagnosed with a Current Episode of an Anxiety or Depressive Disorder: A Meta-Analysis of Randomised Controlled Trials," *PLoS One* 9, no. 4 (Apr. 24, 2014).

428 K. L. Scott et al., "Work-Related Resilience, Engagement and Wellbeing among Music Industry Workers during the COVID-19 Pandemic: A Multiwave Model of Mindfulness and Hope," *Stress Health* 40, no. 5 (2024): e3466.

429 M. K. B. Lustyk et al., "Mindfulness Meditation Research: Issues of Participant Screening, Safety Procedures, and Researcher Training," *Adv Mind Body Med* 24, no. 1 (2009): 20–30.

430 U. Jonsson et al., "Reporting of Harms in Randomized Controlled Trials of Psychological Interventions for Mental and Behavioral Disorders: A Review of Current Practice," *Contemp Clin Trials* 38, no. 1 (2014): 1–8.

431 E. L. Garland, S. A. Gaylord, and B. L. Fredrickson, "Positive Reappraisal Mediates the Stress-Reductive Effects of Mindfulness: An Upward Spiral Process," *Mindfulness* 2, no. 1 (Mar. 1, 2011): 59–67.

432 M. De Couck et al., "How Breathing Can Help You Make Better Decisions: Two Studies on the Effects of Breathing Patterns on Heart Rate Variability and Decision-Making in Business Cases," *International Journal of Psychophysiology* 139 (May 2019): 1–9.

433 M. Y. Balban et al., "Brief Structured Respiration Practices Enhance Mood and Reduce Physiological Arousal," *Cell Rep Med* 4, no. 1 (Jan. 17, 2023).

434 J. E. van der Zwan et al., "Physical Activity, Mindfulness Meditation, or Heart Rate Variability Biofeedback for Stress Reduction: A Randomized Controlled Trial," *Applied Psychophysiology Biofeedback* 40, no. 4 (2015): 257–68.

435 S. Dimitrov, E. Hulteng, and S. Hong, "Inflammation and Exercise: Inhibition of Monocytic Intracellular TNF Production by Acute Exercise via β2-Adrenergic Activation," *Brain Behav Immun* 61 (2017): 60–68.

436 C. Harzer and W. Ruch, "The Relationships of Character Strengths with Coping Work-Related Stress, and Job Satisfaction," *Front Psychol* 6 (February 2015).

437 T. Li, W. Duan, and P. Guo, "Character Strengths, Social Anxiety, and Physiological Stress Reactivity," *PeerJ* 5 (2017).

438 H. Littman-Ovadia, S. Lavy, and M. Boiman-Meshita, "When Theory and Research Collide: Examining Correlates of Signature Strengths Use at Work," *J Happiness Stud* 18, no. 2 (Apr. 1, 2017): 527–48.

439 T. Blanchard, T. Kerbeykian, and R. E. McGrath, "Why Are Signature Strengths and Well-Being Related? Tests of Multiple Hypotheses," *J Happiness Stud* 21, no. 6 (Aug. 1, 2020): 2095–114.

440 N. S. Schutte and J. M. Malouff, "The Impact of Signature Character Strengths Interventions: A Meta-Analysis," *J Happiness Stud* 20, no. 4 (Apr. 15, 2019): 1179–96.

441 VIA Institute on Character, "Who Are You at Your Best?" (2024), https://www.viacharacter.org/.

442 L. F. Cunha, L. C. Pellanda, and C. T. Reppold, "Positive Psychology and Gratitude Interventions: A Randomized Clinical Trial," *Front Psychol* 10 (March 2019).

443 Custom Market Insights, "Global Self-Improvement Market 2024–2033" (November 2023).

444 M. Brenan, "Less than Half of Americans 'Very Satisfied' with Own Lives," *Gallup* (2024).

445 Grand View Research, *Personal Development Market Size, Share & Trends Analysis Report* (2023).

446 S. Starker, *Oracle at the Supermarket: The American Preoccupation with Self-Help* (Piscataway, NJ: Transaction Publishers, 2002).

447 R. M. Ryan and E. L. Deci, "Self-Determination Theory and the Facilitation of Intrinsic Motivation, Social Development, and Well-Being," *American Psychologist* 55, no. 1 (2000): 68–78.

448 E. L. Deci and R. M. Ryan, "Self-Determination Theory: A Macrotheory of Human Motivation, Development, and Health," *Canadian Psychology* 49, no. 3 (2008): 182–5.

449 E. L. Deci and R. M. Ryan, "The 'What' and 'Why' of Goal Pursuits: Human Needs and the Self-Determination of Behavior," *Psychological Inquiry* 4 (2000): 227–68.

450 F. Martela and R. M. Ryan, "The Benefits of Benevolence: Basic Psychological Needs, Beneficence, and the Enhancement of Well-Being," *J Pers* 84, no. 6 (Dec. 1, 2016): 750–64.

451 R. M. Ryan, J. H. Bernstein, and K. Warren Brown, "Weekends, Work, and Well-Being: Psychological Need Satisfactions and Day of the Week Effects on Mood, Vitality, and Physical Symptoms," *J Soc Clin Psychol* 29, no. 1 (2010): 95–122.

452 H. T. Reis et al., "Daily Well-Being: The Role of Autonomy, Competence, and Relatedness," *Personality and Social Psychology Bulletin* 26, no. 4 (2000): 419–35.

453 J. L. Burnette et al., "Mind-Sets Matter: A Meta-Analytic Review of Implicit Theories and Self-Regulation," *Psychol Bull* 139, no. 3 (2013): 655–701.

454 A. L. Duckworth et al, "Grit: Perseverance and Passion for Long-Term Goals," *J Pers Soc Psychol* 92, no. 6 (June 2007): 1087–101.

455 A. T. Vazsonyi et al., "To Grit or Not to Grit, That Is the Question!" *J Res Pers* 78 (Feb. 1, 2019): 215–26.

456 J. A. D. Datu, "Beyond Passion and Perseverance: Review and Future Research Initiatives on the Science of Grit," *Front Psychol* 11 (Jan. 27, 2021).

457 M. Alvesson and K. Einola, "Excessive Work Regimes and Functional Stupidity," *German Journal of Human Resource Management* 32, nos. 3–4 (2018): 283–96.

458 T. Curran et al., "The Psychology of Passion: A Meta-Analytical Review of a Decade of Research on Intrapersonal Outcomes," *Motiv Emot* 39, no. 5 (Oct. 15, 2015): 631–55.

459 R. J. Vallerand et al., "Les Passions de l'Âme: On Obsessive and Harmonious Passion," *J Pers Soc Psychol* 85, no. 4 (2003): 756–67.

460 F. L. Rousseau and R. J. Vallerand, "An Examination of the Relationship between Passion and Subjective Well-Being in Older Adults," *Int J Aging Hum Dev* 66, no. 3 (2008): 195–211.

461 J. Carpentier, G. A. Mageau, and R. J. Vallerand, "Ruminations and Flow: Why Do People with a More Harmonious Passion Experience Higher Well-Being?" *J Happiness Stud* 13, no. 3 (June 2012): 501–18.

462 J. Verner-Filion et al., "The Two Roads from Passion to Sport Performance and Psychological Well-Being: The Mediating Role of Need Satisfaction, Deliberate Practice, and Achievement Goals," *Psychol Sport Exerc* 30 (May 1, 2017): 19–29.

463 J. Verner-Filion and R. J. Vallerand, "On the Differential Relationships Involving Perfectionism and Academic Adjustment: The Mediating Role of Passion and Affect," *Learn Individ Differ* 50 (Aug. 1, 2016): 103–13.

464 P. L. Hewitt and G. L. Flett, "Perfectionism in the Self and Social Contexts: Conceptualization, Assessment, and Association with Psychopathology," *J Pers Soc Psychol* 60, no. 3 (1991): 456–70.

465 R. J. Vallerand, "The Role of Passion in Sustainable Psychological Well-Being," *Psychology of Well-Being: Theory, Research and Practice* 2, no. 1 (2012): 1.

466 R. J. Vallerand et al., "On the Role of Passion in Performance," *J Pers* 75, no. 3 (June 2007): 505–33.

467 R. J. Vallerand et al., "Passion and Performance Attainment in Sport," *Psychol Sport Exerc* 9, no. 3 (May 2008): 373–92.

468 N. Carbonneau et al., "The Role of Passion for Teaching in Intrapersonal and Interpersonal Outcomes," *J Educ Psychol* 100, no. 4 (November 2008): 977–87.

469 F. L. Philippe, R. J. Vallerand, and G. L. Lavigne, "Passion Does Make a Difference in People's Lives: A Look at Well-Being in Passionate and Non-Passionate Individuals," *Appl Psychol Health Well Being* 1, no. 1 (March 2009): 3–22.

470 J. P. Tangney, R. F. Baumeister, and A. L. Boone, "High Self-Control Predicts Good Adjustment, Less Pathology, Better Grades, and Interpersonal Success," *J Pers* 72, no. 2 (2004): 271–324.

471 M. S. Hagger and K. Hamilton, "Trait Self-Control as a Determinant of Health Behavior: Recent Advances on Mechanisms and Future Directions for Research," *Curr Opin Psychol* 60 (December 2024).

472 M. S. Hagger, "Self-Regulation: An Important Construct in Health Psychology Research and Practice," *Health Psychol Rev* 4, no. 2 (2010): 57–65.

473 B. M. Galla and A. L. Duckworth, "More than Resisting Temptation: Beneficial Habits Mediate the Relationship between Self-Control and Positive Life Outcomes," *J Pers Soc Psychol* 109, no. 3 (2015): 508–25.

474 M. Inzlicht and B. W. Roberts, "The Fable of State Self-Control," *Current Opinion in Psychology* 58 (2024).

475 D. Linton, "How Marie Kondo Changed Her Mind about Mess: 'I Realised Perfect Order Was Not My Goal—It Was Spending Time with My Kids,'" *Guardian* (Mar. 30, 2024).

476 R. Kivetz and A. Keinan, "Repenting Hyperopia: An Analysis of Self-Control Regrets," *Journal of Consumer Research* 33, no. 2 (September 2006): 273–82.

477 A. Duckworth and J. J. Gross, "Self-Control and Grit: Related but Separable Determinants of Success," *Curr Dir Psychol Sci* 23, no. 5 (Oct. 11, 2014): 319–25.

478 A. Ponnock et al., "Grit and Conscientiousness: Another Jangle Fallacy," *J Res Pers* 89 (Dec. 1, 2020).

479 K. Muenks et al., "How True Is Grit? Assessing Its Relations to High School and College Students' Personality Characteristics, Self-Regulation, Engagement, and Achievement," *J Educ Psychol* 109, no. 5 (2017): 599.

480 A. Abuhassàn and T. C. Bates, "Grit: Distinguishing Effortful Persistence from Conscientiousness," *J Individ Differ* 36, no. 4 (Nov. 1, 2015): 205–14.

481 T. B. Kashdan and J. Rottenberg, "Psychological Flexibility as a Fundamental Aspect of Health," *Clin Psychol Rev* 30, no. 7 (2010): 865–78.

482 G. Dreisbach and K. Fröber, "On How to Be Flexible (or Not): Modulation of the Stability-Flexibility Balance," *Curr Dir Psychol Sci* 28, no. 1 (2019): 3–9.

483 G. M. Lucas et al., "When the Going Gets Tough: Grit Predicts Costly Perseverance," *J Res Pers* 59 (2015): 15–22.

484 T. Åstebro, S. A. Jeffrey, and G. K. Adomdza, "Inventor Perseverance after Being Told to Quit: The Role of Cognitive Biases," *J Behav Decis Mak* 20, no. 3 (2007): 253–72.

485 W. R. Walker, H. Alexander, and K. Aune, "Higher Levels of Grit Are Associated with a Stronger Fading Affect Bias," *Psychol Rep* 123, no. 1 (2020): 124–40.

486 M. Maltz, *Psycho-Cybernetics* (New York: Prentice Hall, 1960).

487 B. Gardner, P. Lally, and J. Wardle, "Making Health Habitual: The Psychology of 'Habit-Formation' and General Practice," *British Journal of General Practice* 62 (2012): 664–6.

488 P. Lally et al., "How Are Habits Formed: Modelling Habit Formation in the Real World," *Eur J Soc Psychol* 40, no. 6 (October 2010): 998–1009.

489 B. Singh, A. Murphy, C. Maher, and A. E. Smith, "Time to Form a Habit: A Systematic Review and Meta-Analysis of Health Behaviour Habit Formation and Its Determinants," *Healthcare (Basel)* 12, no. 23 (December 2024): 2488.

490 A. Buyalskaya et al., "What Can Machine Learning Teach Us about Habit Formation? Evidence from Exercise and Hygiene," *PNAS* 120 (2023).

491 M. Gladwell, *Outliers: The Story of Success* (London: Penguin, 2008).

492 K. A. Ericsson, R. T. Krampe, and C. Tesch-Roemer, "The Role of Deliberate Practice in the Acquisition of Expert Performance," *Psychol Rev* 100, no. 3 (1993): 363–406.

493 K. A. Ericsson, "The Danger of Delegating Education to Journalists" (2012).

494 B. N. Macnamara, D. Z. Hambrick, and F. L. Oswald, "Deliberate Practice and Performance in Music, Games, Sports, Education, and Professions: A Meta-Analysis," *Psychol Sci* 25, no. 8 (2014): 1608–18.

495 B. N. Macnamara, D. Moreau, and D. Z. Hambrick, "The Relationship between Deliberate Practice and Performance in Sports: A Meta-Analysis," *Perspectives on Psychological Science* 11, no. 3 (May 1, 2016): 333–50.

496 R. M. Ryan and J. H. Lynch, "Emotional Autonomy versus Detachment: Revisiting the Vicissitudes of Adolescence and Young Adulthood," *Child Dev* 60 (1989): 340–56.

497 R. M. Ryan, J. D. Stiller, and J. H. Lynch, "Representations of Relationships to Teachers, Parents, and Friends as Predictors of Academic Motivation and Self-Esteem," *J Early Adolesc* 14, no. 2 (1994): 226–49.

498 Y. Kim, J. S. Butzel, and R. M. Ryan, "Interdependence and Well-Being: A Function of Culture and Relatedness Needs," in *International Society for the Study of Personal Relationships* (Saratoga Springs, NY, 1998).

499 S. Buecker et al., "Is Loneliness in Emerging Adults Increasing Over Time? A Preregistered Cross-Temporal Meta-Analysis and Systematic Review," *Psychol Bull* 147, no. 8 (2021): 787–805.

500 I. Goddard, "What Does Friendship Look Like in America?" (October 2023).

501 Office of the Surgeon General, "Our Epidemic of Loneliness and Isolation: The US Surgeon General's Advisory on the Healing Effects of Social Connection and Community" (2023).

502 Kadence, "Younger Workers Fear Loneliness from Long-Term Home Working" (September 2021).

503 F. Mann et al., "Loneliness and the Onset of New Mental Health Problems in the General Population," *Social Psychiatry and Psychiatric Epidemiology* 57 (2022): 2161–78.

504 M. E. Loades et al., "Rapid Systematic Review: The Impact of Social Isolation and Loneliness on the Mental Health of Children and Adolescents in the Context of COVID-19," *J Am Acad Child Adolesc Psychiatry* 59 (2020), https://www.jaacap.org.

505 C. D. Shepherd et al., "Entrepreneurial Burnout: Exploring Antecedents, Dimensions and Outcomes," *Journal of Research in Marketing and Entrepreneurship* 12, no. 1 (2010): 71–9.

506 J. Forest et al., "Harmonious Passion as an Explanation of the Relation between Signature Strengths' Use and Well-Being at Work: Test of an Intervention Program," *Human Relations* 65, no. 9 (2012): 1233–52.

507 T. Curran and A. P. Hill, "Perfectionism Is Increasing Over Time: A Meta-Analysis of Birth Cohort Differences from 1989 to 2016," *Psychol Bull* 145, no. 4 (Apr. 1, 2019): 410–29.

508 M. Ferrari et al., "Self-Compassion Moderates the Perfectionism and Depression Link in Both Adolescence and Adulthood," *PLoS One* 13, no. 2 (Feb. 21, 2018).

509 W. J. Phillips and D. W. Hine, "Self-Compassion, Physical Health, and Health Behaviour: A Meta-Analysis," *Health Psychol Rev* 15, no. 1 (2021): 113–39.

510 R. F. Baumeister et al., "Ego Depletion: Is the Active Self a Limited Resource?" *J Pers Soc Psychol* 74, no. 5 (1998): 1252–65.

511 E. T. Berkman et al., "Self-Control as Value-Based Choice," *Curr Dir Psychol Sci* 26, no. 5 (Oct. 1, 2017): 422–8.

512 M. Inzlicht et al., "Integrating Models of Self-Regulation," *Annu Rev Psychol* 72 (2021): 319–45.

513 M. Milyavskaya and M. Inzlicht, "What's So Great about Self-Control? Examining the Importance of Effortful Self-Control and Temptation in Predicting Real-Life Depletion and Goal Attainment," *Soc Psychol Personal Sci* 8, no. 6 (Aug. 1, 2017): 603–11.

514 M. Quirin, M. Tops, and J. Kuhl, "Autonomous Motivation, Internalization, and the Self: A Functional Approach of Interacting Neuropsychological Systems," in *The Oxford Handbook of Human Motivation*, 2nd ed., ed. R. M. Ryan (Oxford: Oxford University Press, 2019), 393–414.

515 W. Lee and J. Reeve, "Motivational Neuroscience," in *The Oxford Handbook of Human Motivation*, ed. R. M. Ryan (Oxford: Oxford University Press, 2019), 354–72.

516 M. L. Scott and S. M. Nowlis, "The Effect of Goal Specificity on Consumer Goal Reengagement," *Journal of Consumer Research* 40, no. 3 (October 2013): 444–59.

517 J. Reeve and W. Lee, "Neuroscience and Human Motivation," in *The Oxford Handbook of Human Motivation*, ed. R. M. Ryan (Oxford: Oxford University Press, 2012), 365–80.

518 A. C. Holding and R. Koestner, "The Role of Motivation in the Lifecycle of Personal Goals," in *The Oxford Handbook of Self-Determination Theory*, ed. R. M. Ryan (Oxford: Oxford Academic, 2023), 327–45.

519 O. Williamson et al., "The Performance and Psychological Effects of Goal Setting in Sport: A Systematic Review and Meta-Analysis," *Int Rev Sport Exerc Psychol* 17, no. 2 (2022): 1050–78.

520 J. P. Millonado Valdez and J. A. Daep Datu, "How Do Grit and Gratitude Relate to Flourishing? The Mediating Role of Emotion Regulation," in *Multidisciplinary Perspectives on Grit: Contemporary Theories, Assessments, Applications and Critiques*, eds. L. E. van Zyle, C. Olckers, and L. van der Vaart (Cham: Springer Nature, 2021), 1–16.

521 A. Duke, *Quit: The Power of Knowing When to Walk Away* (London: Ebury Edge, 2022).

522 J. A. Hall et al., "Quality Conversation Can Increase Daily Well-Being," *Communic Res* 52, no. 3 (Jan. 27, 2023).

523 N. Weinstein, A. K. Przybylski, and R. M. Ryan, "Can Nature Make Us More Caring? Effects of Immersion in Nature on Intrinsic Aspirations and Generosity," *Pers Soc Psychol Bull* 35, no. 10 (October 2009): 1315–29.

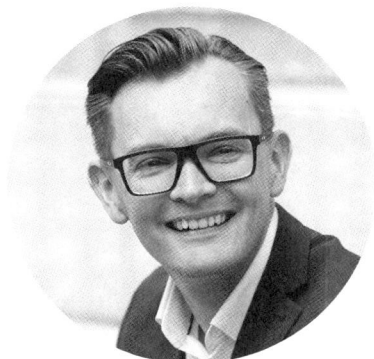

ABOUT THE AUTHOR

Dr. James Hewitt combines rigorous science with real-world experience to revolutionize how we think about performance. A former full-time racing cyclist turned human performance scientist, he founded The Knowledge Work Lab to help organizations thrive in an always-on world. James's research, consulting, and keynote speaking have impacted organizations in over thirty countries, from Fortune 500 boardrooms to Formula One paddocks. James helps leaders and teams move beyond optimization to embrace regenerative performance, enabling them to achieve extraordinary results without sacrificing well-being.